CASE REVIEW
Thoracic Imaging

Series Editor

David M. Yousem, MD
Professor, Department of Radiology
Director of Neuroradiology
Johns Hopkins Hospital
Baltimore, Maryland

Other Volumes in the CASE REVIEW Series

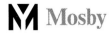

Mosby

An Imprint of Elsevier Science

St. Louis London Philadelphia Sydney Toronto

Phillip M. Boiselle, MD
Director of Thoracic Imaging
Beth Israel Deaconess Medical Center
Assistant Professor of Radiology
Harvard Medical School
Boston, Massachusetts

Theresa C. McLoud, MD
Director of Thoracic and Cardiac Radiology
Associate Radiologist-in-Chief
Director of Education
Massachusetts General Hospital
Professor of Radiology
Harvard Medical School
Boston, Massachusetts

WITH 276 ILLUSTRATIONS

CASE REVIEW

Thoracic Imaging

CASE REVIEW SERIES

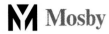

Mosby

An Imprint of Elsevier Science

Acquisitions Editor: Stephanie Donley
Project Manager: Agnes Hunt Byrne
Production Manager: Peter Faber
Illustration Specialist: Robert Quinn
Indexer: Dennis Dolan

Mosby, Inc.
An Imprint of Elsevier Science
11830 Westline Industrial Drive
St. Louis, Missouri 63146

Printed in the United States of America.

International Standard Book Number 0–323–00656–6

Library of Congress Cataloging-in-Publication Data

Boiselle, Phillip M.
Thoracic imaging: case review / Phillip M. Boiselle, Theresa McLoud.

p.   cm.

ISBN 0–323–00656–6

1. Chest—Imaging—Case studies.   2. Chest—Diseases—Diagnosis—Case
   studies.   I. McLoud, Theresa C.   II. Title.
   [DNLM: 1. Thoracic Diseases—diagnosis—Case Report.   2. Diagnostic
   Imaging—Case Report.   WF 975 B682t 2001]

RC941.B67 2001   617.5′40754—dc21   00–048044

Last digit is the print number: 9   8   7   6   5   4   3   2

To my wife, Ellen
PMB

To my sister, Veronica
TCM

In most institutions, residency training begins with the analysis of the chest radiograph. It takes months of study before this simple yet elegant examination is mastered. Then, just when you think you are proficient in diagnosing pulmonary pathology, you are introduced to chest computed tomography and suddenly you realize just how much you are **not** seeing on the plain chest x-ray. With high resolution chest computed tomography and pulmonary angiography, the bar gets raised even further. To truly excel as a chest radiologist you must understand both the tools at your disposal and the implications of the pathology in question.

In Phil Boiselle and Theresa McLoud you have two such outstanding chest radiologists and teachers. They have contributed a wonderful addition to the Case Review Series, a series designed to review each specialty in a challenging, interactive way. Each book in the series has gradations of difficulty so that the reader can assess his or her proficiency and can use this self-evaluation to guide continued education. By referencing THE REQUISITES textbook, the reader can "bone up" on a topic if a weakness is perceived. Since each case in the book is distinct, this is the kind of text that you can pick up and review at any time in your day or in your career.

Drs. Boiselle and McLoud have written a fantastic book that I recommend for all radiologists and clinicians who examine the chest.

David M. Yousem, MD

The presentation and discussion of "unknown" cases is an integral component of formal diagnostic radiology education. The Case Review series uses this established format as a means of providing focused, subspecialty examination preparation for radiology residents. This book, *Thoracic Imaging*, will likely also serve as a practical review for fellows and practicing radiologists who wish to sharpen their skills in this area.

The primary goals of this book are twofold. First, to use a case format presentation to illustrate and review the imaging features of disorders that span the spectrum of thoracic diseases with which a graduating resident should have a working familiarity. Accordingly, *Thoracic Imaging* comprises a diverse group of 150 cases using images from several modalities, including conventional radiography, computed tomography, high-resolution computed tomography, and magnetic resonance imaging. Similar to books in this series, the cases are categorized by level of difficulty: Opening Round, Fair Game, and Challenge. Each case is followed by a list of questions, with answers provided on the verso page. The answers are followed by a brief discussion section that emphasizes characteristic imaging features, differential diagnostic considerations, and key points of clinical information for each case. For readers who desire additional information about a given topic, we have included a helpful reference for further reading. A cross-reference to *Thoracic Radiology: THE REQUISITES* is also provided.

Second, it is our goal to help the reader to develop a sound framework with which to approach image interpretation in thoracic radiology. As teachers of radiology, we place dual emphasis on methodology and final diagnosis, believing that the means by which one reaches the final diagnosis is as important as arriving at a correct answer. Indeed, for some of the cases in this book, a specific, correct diagnosis is not expected from the reader.

This book is a collaborative project that has benefitted from the help of many. We are especially grateful to: Stephanie Donley, our editor at Harcourt Health Sciences, for editorial assistance; Dr. David Yousem, the editor of this series, for support and guidance; Nancy Williams, for administrative assistance; Dr. Ferris Hall, for contributing several cases; and Milne Hewish, for photography.

We hope that *Thoracic Imaging* will prove a valuable learning tool for its readers.

Phillip M. Boiselle, MD
Theresa C. McLoud, MD

Opening Round

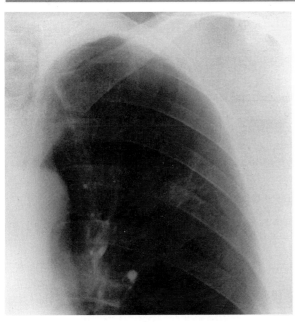 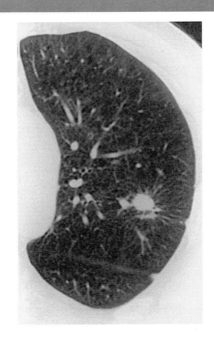

1. Which imaging feature of this nodule is of concern for malignancy?
2. Which cell type of lung cancer is most likely?
3. What is the size criteria for a T1 lesion?
4. Is this lesion better suited to image-guided transthoracic needle biopsy or bronchoscopic biopsy?

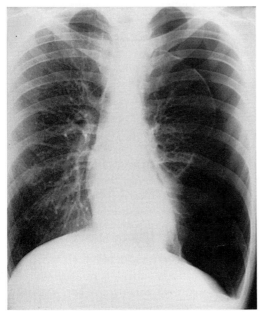 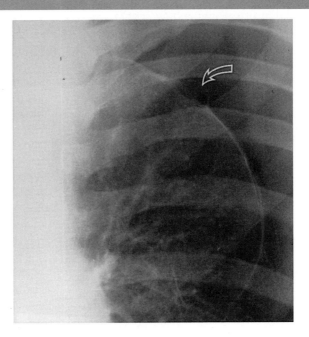

1. What is the cause of this patient's pleuritic chest pain and dyspnea?
2. Name at least five causes of pneumothorax.
3. Based on the imaging findings in this case, what is the most likely cause for this "spontaneous" pneumothorax?
4. What radiographic finding(s) in this case suggests the possibility of a tension pneumothorax?

CASE 1

Bronchogenic Carcinoma

1. Spiculated margins.

2. Adenocarcinoma.

3. Less than 3 cm in diameter.

4. Transthoracic needle biopsy.

Reference

Jett J, Feins R, Kvale P, et al: Pretreatment evaluation of non-small cell lung cancer. *Am J Respir Crit Care Med* 156:320–332, 1997.

Cross-Reference

Thoracic Radiology: THE REQUISITES, pp 340–343.

Comment

A solitary pulmonary nodule is defined as a well-circumscribed round or oval lesion measuring less than 3 cm in diameter. There are only two specific and reliable signs of benignity on chest radiographs: (1) identification of a benign pattern of calcification or (2) demonstration of absolute absence of growth over a 2-year period. For cases that do not meet one of these criteria, thin-section CT is generally recommended for further evaluation. In comparison with radiography, CT allows a more accurate assessment of the margins of a nodule; moreover, CT is more sensitive for identifying the presence and distribution of calcium and fat within a nodule.

The nodule in this case has spiculated margins, a finding that is highly suspicious for malignancy. Depending on local practice patterns and clinical circumstances, a preoperative biopsy may be requested. The peripheral location of this nodule makes it best suited for a transthoracic needle biopsy.

The most common cell type of lung cancer is adenocarcinoma. It most often presents as a solitary, peripheral nodule with spiculated margins. Based on size criteria, this is a T1 lesion. A T1 lesion is defined as a nodule that is less than 3 cm in diameter and completely surrounded by lung or visceral pleura. Such lesions have a relatively favorable prognosis (approximately 70% 5-year survival) when there is no evidence of nodal or distant metastases.

Notes

CASE 2

Spontaneous Pneumothorax Secondary to Ruptured Bleb

1. Pneumothorax.

2. Spontaneous, chronic obstructive pulmonary disease, chronic infiltrative lung disease (e.g., histiocytosis X and lymphangioleiomyomatosis), malignant neoplasms (e.g., metastatic sarcoma), trauma, catamenial pneumothorax, iatrogenic, barotrauma, and infection (e.g., lung abscess and septic infarcts).

3. Ruptured apical bleb.

4. Depression of the left hemidiaphragm; expansion of the left rib cage.

Reference

Wilson AG: Pleura and pleural disorders. In: Armstrong P, Wilson AG, Dee P, Hansell DM, Eds: *Imaging of Diseases of the Chest*, second edition. St. Louis, Mosby, 1995, pp 690–700.

Cross-Reference

Thoracic Radiology: THE REQUISITES, pp 496–501.

Comment

Pneumothorax is defined as the presence of air or gas within the pleural space. Although there are a wide variety of causes, spontaneous pneumothorax is the most common etiology. Affected patients are usually in the third or fourth decade of life.

Spontaneous pneumothoraces are almost always secondary to rupture of an apical bleb, which represents a gas pocket within the elastic fibers of the visceral pleura. Note the presence of a small bleb along the visceral pleural margin in this patient, which is best demonstrated on the coned-down image of the left upper lobe (*arrow*, second figure). Such blebs have been reported to be detectable on chest radiographs in approximately 15% of cases of spontaneous pneumothorax. However, blebs are rarely evident on radiographs following resolution of the pneumothorax. CT is much more sensitive than radiography for detecting blebs. It has been shown to detect blebs in approximately 80% of patients following resolution of spontaneous pneumothoraces. The size and number of apical blebs detected on CT have been shown to correlate with the risk of recurrent pneumothoraces and the need for surgical intervention.

Tension pneumothorax is a life-threatening condition that presents with clinical signs of tachypnea, tachycardia, cyanosis, sweating, and hypotension. Radiographic findings may include contralateral mediastinal shift, diaphragmatic depression, rib cage expansion, and flattening of the contours of the right heart border and/or vena cavae.

Notes

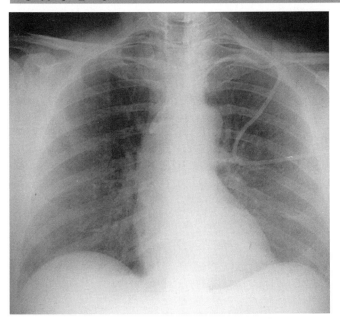 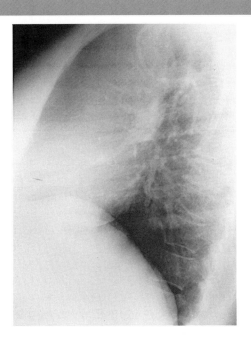

1. Where is this central venous catheter located?
2. Should the catheter be repositioned?
3. What is the most common complication of inadvertent placement of a catheter in this location?
4. Is inadvertent azygos vein cannulation more common following a left- or right-sided vascular insertion approach?

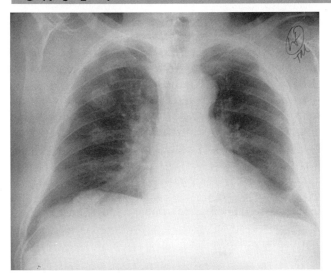 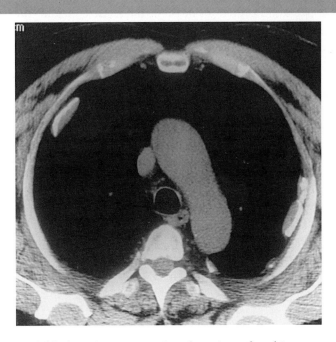

1. Based on the imaging findings in this case, name several likely prior occupational settings for this individual.
2. Are pleural plaques from prior asbestos exposure usually unilateral or bilateral?
3. Are these lesions symptomatic?
4. Are pleural plaques premalignant?

CASE 3

Malpositioned Catheter in the Azygos Vein

1. Azygos vein.

2. Yes.

3. Venous rupture.

4. Left-sided.

Reference

Bankier AA, Reinhold M, Weismayr MN, et al: Azygos arch cannulation by central venous catheters: radiographic detection of malposition and subsequent complications. *J Thorac Imaging* 12:64-69; 1997.

Cross-Reference

Thoracic Radiology: THE REQUISITES, pp 154-159.

Comment

Inadvertent insertion of a catheter into the azygos vein is a relatively uncommon complication of central venous catheter placement, with an estimated frequency of approximately 1%. Detection of a malpositioned catheter at this site is important, because there is a relatively high frequency of associated venous perforation.

Note the abnormal curve of the catheter at the level of the azygos arch on the posteroanterior (PA) chest radiograph. The precise location is confirmed on the lateral chest radiograph (second figure), which demonstrates the posterior course of the catheter within the azygos arch.

Interestingly, azygos vein cannulation occurs most commonly following left-sided catheter insertion. This association is thought to occur secondary to anterocaudal arching of the left brachiocephalic vein, which may preferentially promote entry of a catheter into the azygos vein rather than the superior vena cava. In contrast, catheters placed from the right side of the thorax have a more direct course to the superior vena cava via the right brachiocephalic vein.

Notes

CASE 4

Calcified Pleural Plaques From Prior Asbestos Exposure

1. Mining, insulation manufacturing, textile manufacturing, construction, ship building, and brake lining manufacturing and repair.

2. Bilateral.

3. No.

4. No.

Reference

McLoud TC: Conventional radiography in the diagnosis of asbestos-related disease. *Radiol Clin North Am* 30:1177-1189, 1992.

Cross-Reference

Thoracic Radiology: THE REQUISITES, pp 234-238.

Comment

The chest radiograph demonstrates numerous calcified lesions bilaterally, several of which are plateau-like in configuration and parallel the inner margin of the lateral thoracic wall. The CT image confirms the pleural location of these lesions and demonstrates the calcification to a better degree. The appearance is typical of pleural plaques related to prior asbestos exposure.

Pleural plaques are the most common manifestation of asbestos exposure. Such plaques typically occur after an approximately 20-year latency period. They are asymptomatic and usually discovered incidentally. Pathologically, pleural plaques are composed of dense bands of avascular collagen, and they are not considered premalignant.

The chest radiographic appearance is dependent on whether a plaque is seen in profile or en face. When observed in profile, a plaque appears as a dense band of soft tissue opacity paralleling the inner margin of the lateral thoracic wall. When observed en face, a plaque appears as a veil-like opacity with irregular edges, often described as a "holly leaf" configuration. Plaques are usually bilateral and often symmetric. The lower half of the thorax is most often affected, usually between the sixth and ninth ribs.

Notes

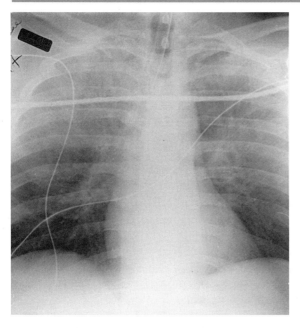
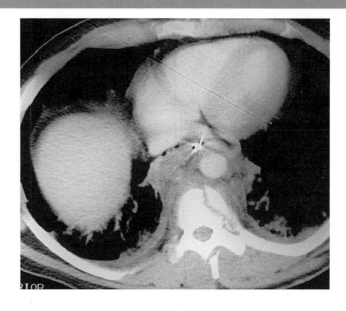

1. Displacement of the paraspinal lines implies an abnormality in which mediastinal compartment?
2. Are thoracic vertebral body fractures commonly associated with mediastinal hematoma?
3. How reliable are portable chest radiographs for detecting spinal fractures?
4. Which portion of the spine is most susceptible to traumatic injury?

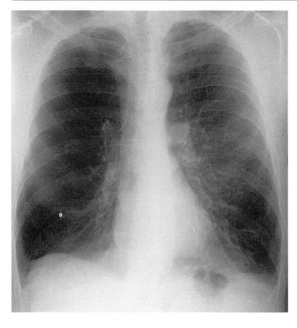
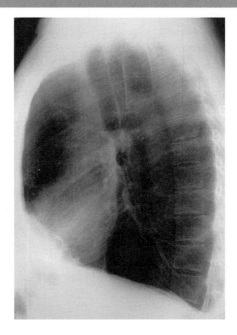

1. What are the two major chest radiographic features of emphysema?
2. What is the best chest radiographic indicator of overinflation of the lungs?
3. Is the chest radiograph a reliable tool for detecting emphysema?
4. What is the most sensitive imaging modality for detecting emphysema?

C A S E 5

Vertebral Body Fracture With Paraspinal Hematoma

1. Posterior.

2. Yes.

3. Not very reliable.

4. The thoracolumbar junction (T-12–L-2).

Reference

Kuhlman JE, Pozniak MA, Collins J, Knisely BL: Radiographic and CT findings of blunt chest trauma: aortic injuries and looking beyond them. *Radiographics* 18:1085-1106, 1998.

Cross-Reference

Thoracic Radiology: THE REQUISITES, pp 177-179, 423.

Comment

Thoracic spine fracture is an infrequent but serious complication of blunt trauma. Unfortunately, the portable trauma chest radiograph is not very reliable in detecting spinal fractures. In fact, it has been reported that only approximately 50% of spinal fractures can be identified at initial chest radiography!

Radiographic findings associated with spinal fracture include findings related to mediastinal hemorrhage (such as widening of the paraspinal lines, mediastinal widening, and left apical pleural cap) and vertebral abnormalities. The latter are more specific for spinal injury and include loss of height of the vertebral body and obscuration of the pedicle(s). When you identify a mediastinal hematoma that is confined to the posterior mediastinum, you should diligently search for evidence of a vertebral body fracture. If a spinal fracture is not evident on chest radiography, additional imaging with dedicated spine films or CT may be helpful to identify and characterize the fracture.

Notes

C A S E 6

Emphysema

1. Overinflation of the lungs and reduced vascularity.

2. Flattening of the hemidiaphragms.

3. No.

4. High-resolution CT (HRCT) of the chest.

Reference

Webb WR: Radiology of obstructive pulmonary disease. *AJR Am J Roentgenol* 169:637-647, 1997.

Cross-Reference

Thoracic Radiology: THE REQUISITES, pp 287-295.

Comment

Emphysema is defined as permanent, abnormal enlargement of airspaces distal to the terminal bronchiole, accompanied by destruction of their walls.

Radiographic abnormalities in patients with emphysema are related to overinflation of the lungs and lung destruction. The latter is characterized by reduced vascularity or the presence of bullae. Overinflation of the lungs may be characterized by a number of findings, most notably flattening of the hemidiaphragms and an increase in the retrosternal airspace diameter.

Chest radiographic abnormalities are usually evident in moderate to severe cases of emphysema, but radiographs are frequently normal in patients with early emphysema. Chest HRCT is superior to chest radiographs in detecting and characterizing emphysema. This modality has high sensitivity and specificity for the diagnosis of emphysema.

Notes

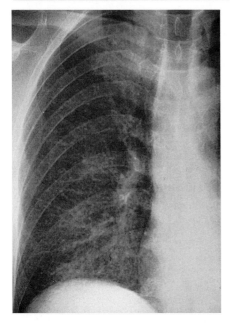
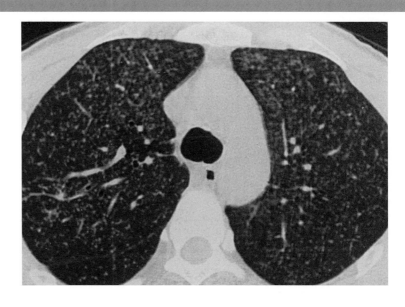

1. What infection is most commonly associated with this pattern?
2. In cases of miliary tuberculosis (TB), how is the infection disseminated to the lung?
3. What other type of infection commonly presents with a miliary pattern?
4. Name four noninfectious entities that may present with a miliary pattern.

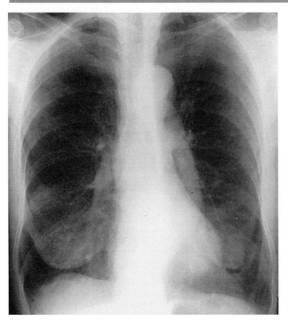
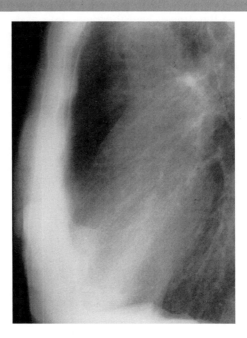

1. Where are the nodular opacities located?
2. What imaging feature on the PA radiograph suggests this location?
3. What is the most common chest wall structure to appear as a nodular opacity on a chest radiograph?
4. How can you confirm a suspected cutaneous site of a nodular opacity using chest radiography?

Miliary Tuberculosis

1. Miliary TB.

2. Hematogenously.

3. Fungal infection.

4. Pneumoconioses (e.g., silicosis), eosinophilic granuloma, sarcoidosis, and metastases (e.g., thyroid, melanoma).

Reference

Reed JC: Diffuse fine nodular disease. In: *Chest Radiology: Plain Film Patterns and Differential Diagnoses*, fourth edition. St. Louis, Mosby–Year Book, 1997, pp 280–294.

Cross-Reference

Thoracic Radiology: THE REQUISITES, pp 33–35, 119, 120, 203.

Comment

A miliary pattern refers to the presence of numerous small (approximately 1- to 2-mm-diameter) lung nodules. Such nodules are difficult to detect radiographically because of their small size. It has been suggested that these tiny nodules become visible radiographically because of the effect of summation.

The classic entity associated with this pattern is miliary TB, which refers to the diffuse hematogenous dissemination of TB. This pattern typically occurs in patients with altered host resistance to the primary infection. Affected patients usually present with fever, chills, and night sweats.

Because of the small size of miliary nodules, it is not surprising that CT (particularly HRCT) is more sensitive than radiography for detection. In fact, it has been estimated that it may take up to 6 weeks for miliary nodules to become apparent on chest radiographs! On HRCT, the nodules are shown to be diffuse and random in distribution.

Notes

Neurofibromas

1. Chest wall.

2. Incomplete, sharp borders.

3. The nipples.

4. Repeat the radiograph with a small lead marker on the site of the cutaneous abnormality.

Reference

Reed JC: Chest wall lesions. In: *Chest Radiology: Plain Film Patterns and Differential Diagnoses*, fourth edition. St. Louis, Mosby–Year Book, 1997, pp 6–21.

Cross-Reference

Thoracic Radiology: THE REQUISITES, pp 48–49.

Comment

When visible on chest radiographs, cutaneous chest wall lesions such as neurofibromas, moles, and nipples demonstrate a characteristic incomplete, sharp border. The sharp border is produced by the interface of the lesion with adjacent air, and it becomes incomplete where the lesion is continuous with the soft tissues of the chest wall. The identification of such a border is helpful for differentiating chest wall lesions from intrapulmonary lesions.

In this particular case, the cutaneous location of the nodules is easily confirmed on the lateral projection. When in doubt about a possible cutaneous location of a focal nodular opacity, one should perform a repeat radiograph with small lead markers for confirmation.

Notes

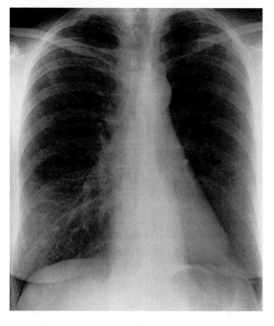
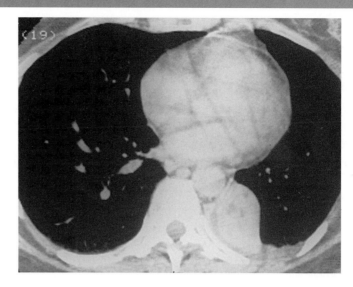

1. What is the diagnosis?
2. Name two primary signs of atelectasis.
3. Name five secondary signs of atelectasis.
4. What is the most common mechanism for complete lobar collapse?

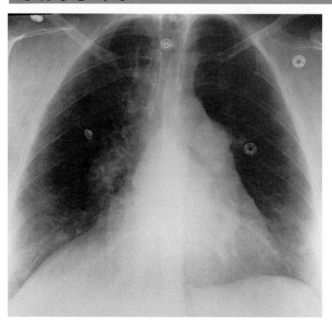
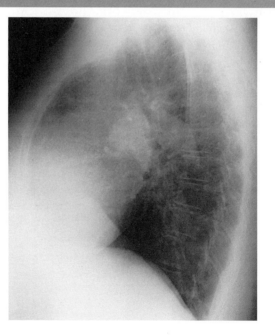

1. What disorder of pulmonary vascularity is evident in this case?
2. What is the difference between primary and secondary pulmonary artery hypertension (PAH)?
3. Is primary PAH more common in men or women?
4. Does a normal chest radiograph exclude the diagnosis of PAH?

CASE 9

Complete Left Lower Lobe Atelectasis

1. Complete left lower lobe atelectasis.

2. Opacification of the affected lobe and displacement of the interlobar fissures.

3. Elevation of the hemidiaphragm, mediastinal shift, displacement of the hilum, compensatory hyperinflation, and crowded vessels.

4. Obstruction of a central bronchus.

Reference

Woodring JH, Reed JC: Radiographic manifestations of lobar atelectasis. *J Thorac Imaging* 11:109-144, 1996.

Cross-Reference

Thoracic Radiology: THE REQUISITES, pp 35-48.

Comment

Atelectasis is defined as a decrease in volume of all or a portion of the lung. The most common type of atelectasis occurs secondary to obstruction of a central bronchus. It is referred to as resorption atelectasis and usually involves an entire lobe.

The chest radiograph and CT image reveal the classic features of complete left lower lobe atelectasis. On chest radiographs, complete left lower lobe atelectasis appears as a triangular opacity behind the heart. The displaced major fissure is seen as an interface between the opacified atelectatic lobe and the hyperexpanded left upper lobe. Note the presence of several secondary signs of atelectasis in this case, including inferomedial displacement of the left hilum, slight leftward shift of the mediastinum, and compensatory hyperinflation of the left upper lobe.

In an outpatient setting, the presence of lobar collapse is usually indicative of an obstructing central mass. In an adult patient, bronchogenic carcinoma and carcinoid are important diagnostic considerations. In a child, an aspirated foreign body is the most likely diagnosis. CT is helpful for identifying the centrally obstructing lesion and for guiding bronchoscopic procedures.

Notes

CASE 10

Primary Pulmonary Artery Hypertension

1. Pulmonary artery hypertension (PAH).

2. In secondary PAH, the hypertension has a known cause; in primary PAH, the cause is unknown.

3. Women.

4. No.

Reference

Rubin LJ: Primary pulmonary hypertension. *N Engl J Med* 336:111-117, 1997.

Cross-Reference

Thoracic Radiology: THE REQUISITES, pp 403-407.

Comment

PAH is defined as a condition of sustained elevation of pulmonary artery pressure. PAH may occur secondary to one of three basic mechanisms: (1) increased pulmonary blood flow (e.g., left-to-right shunt), (2) decreased cross-sectional area of the pulmonary vasculature (e.g., chronic pulmonary embolism), and (3) increased resistance to pulmonary venous drainage (e.g., mitral valve disease).

The majority of cases of PAH occur secondary to a known cause. These cases are collectively referred to as secondary PAH. In a minority of cases, the etiology of PAH remains unknown. These cases are referred to as primary PAH. This condition tends to affect women younger than 40 years of age.

Regardless of the type of PAH, the characteristic findings on chest radiographs are similar. There is usually marked enlargement of the main and hilar pulmonary arteries, which rapidly taper as they course distally. The degree of pulmonary artery enlargement varies considerably, and significant PAH can be present in the setting of a normal chest radiograph. CT is more accurate than chest radiography for detecting pulmonary artery enlargement.

Notes

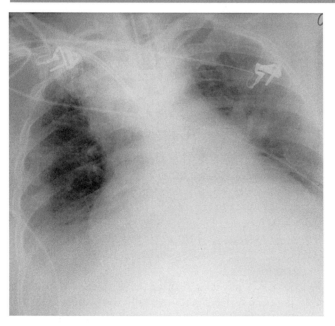
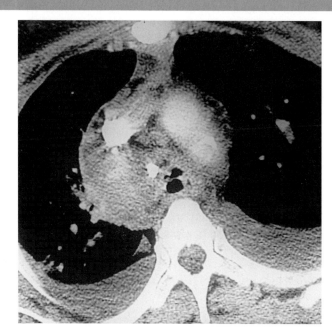

1. What is the most likely cause of mediastinal hematoma in this patient?
2. What is the most common complication of central catheter placement?
3. What is the optimal location for a central venous catheter?
4. Name two complications associated with catheter placement in the right atrium.

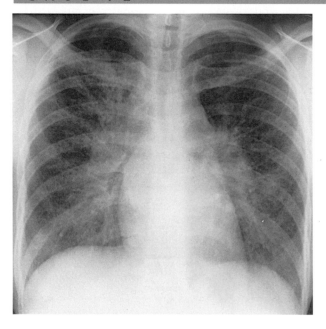
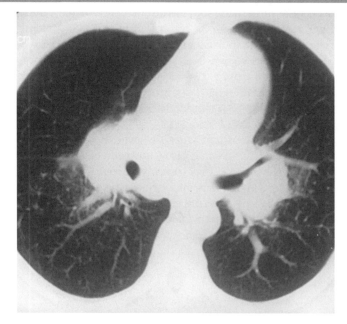

1. What is the most common cause of bilateral, symmetric hilar lymph node enlargement?
2. What percentage of sarcoid patients with hilar lymphadenopathy also have lung parenchymal disease?
3. What percentage of patients with sarcoidosis are asymptomatic at the initial presentation?
4. Are noncaseating granulomas specific for sarcoidosis?

Mediastinal Hematoma Secondary to Vascular Perforation by a Central Venous Catheter

1. Vascular perforation by central venous catheter.

2. Malposition.

3. The superior vena cava.

4. Arrhythmia and cardiac perforation.

Reference

Kidney DD, Deutsch LS: Misplaced central venous catheters: venous anatomy, clinical significance, and treatment options. *Radiologist* 5:119–126, 1998.

Cross-Reference

Thoracic Radiology: THE REQUISITES, pp 154–159.

Comment

The most common complication of central venous catheter placement is malposition, which occurs in up to 40% of cases. Pneumothorax is the second most common complication, occurring in approximately 5% of cases. Less common complications include hemothorax, extrapleural hematoma, cardiac arrhythmias, vascular or cardiac perforation, peripheral venous thrombosis, catheter fragmentation, septic emboli, and mycotic aneurysms. Interventional radiologists are playing an increasingly prominent role in catheter placement. They have a high success rate and a low complication rate, reflecting their expertise in vascular catheterization.

Because of its high flow rate and large volume, the superior vena cava is the ideal location for a central venous catheter. The distal portion of the catheter should lie parallel to the direction of blood flow, and it should not abut the vessel wall.

Catheter malposition is usually evident on a frontal chest radiograph. In some cases, however, a lateral view is necessary to determine the precise location of the catheter tip. In a small minority of cases, a contrast study is necessary to verify catheter location.

In this case, note the unusual medial course of the catheter on the chest radiograph. The CT image confirms an extravascular location.

Notes

Sarcoid

1. Sarcoidosis.

2. Approximately 50%.

3. Approximately 50%.

4. No.

Reference

Miller BH, Rosado-de-Christenson ML, McAdams HP, Fishback NF: Thoracic sarcoidosis: radiologic-pathologic correlation. *Radiographics* 15:421–437, 1995.

Cross-Reference

Thoracic Radiology: THE REQUISITES, pp 213 –216.

Comment

Sarcoidosis is a systemic disorder of unknown etiology that is characterized pathologically by widespread non-caseating granulomas. Because this pathologic finding may also be seen in a variety of other conditions, a diagnosis of sarcoidosis requires consistent radiologic, clinical, laboratory, and pathologic findings, as well as exclusion of other entities (especially granulomatous infections).

The chest radiograph is abnormal in approximately 90% of patients with sarcoid. Bilateral, symmetric hilar lymph node enlargement is the most common radiographic abnormality. It is frequently accompanied by mediastinal lymph node enlargement. Lung parenchymal disease is usually nodular or reticulonodular in appearance, with a predilection for the upper lung zones.

On CT examination (particularly HRCT), sarcoid granulomas typically appear as small (1- to 2-mm-diameter) nodules, with a characteristic perilymphatic distribution. This distribution includes the peribronchovascular lymphatics (second figure), the interlobular septa, and the subpleural lymphatics (peripherally and along the fissures). Approximately 20% of patients with radiographic evidence of interstitial lung disease develop interstitial fibrosis.

Notes

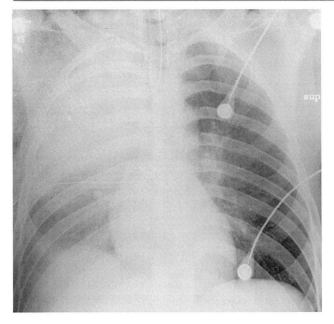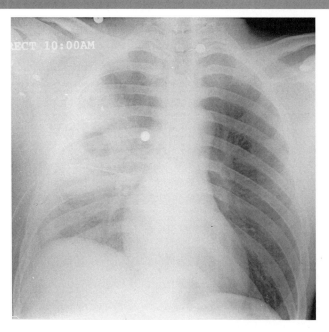

1. What is the most likely cause of parenchymal opacification in this patient who recently sustained a gunshot injury to the right hemithorax?

2. Is contusion an early or late sign of thoracic trauma?

3. When would you expect a contusion to resolve?

4. What other parenchymal injury is evident on the second radiograph of this patient?

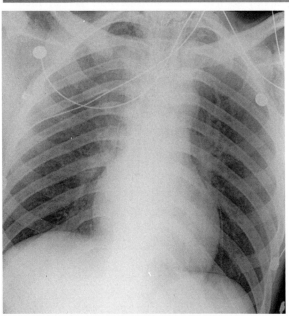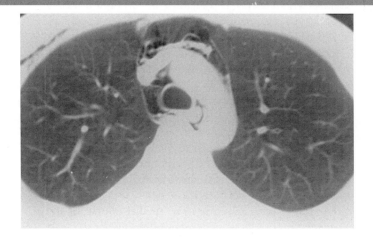

1. Name the location of the intrathoracic, extraalveolar air collection that is evident on the radiograph and CT image.

2. Is there another intrathoracic, extraalveolar air collection evident on the radiograph?

3. What is the most common mechanism for the development of pneumomediastinum?

4. Would you expect pneumomediastinum to change in configuration on a decubitus radiograph?

Pulmonary Contusion and Laceration

1. Pulmonary contusion.

2. Early (within 6 hours).

3. Within 7 days.

4. Pulmonary laceration.

Reference

Kuhlman JE, Pozniak MA, Collins J, Knisely BL: Radiographic and CT findings of blunt chest trauma: aortic injuries and looking beyond them. *Radiographics* 18:1085–1106, 1998.

Cross-Reference

Thoracic Radiology: THE REQUISITES, p 184.

Comment

Thoracic trauma may result in two forms of lung parenchymal injury: pulmonary contusion and pulmonary laceration. Pulmonary contusion is the most common form of lung injury and represents hemorrhage into the alveoli. On radiographs, pulmonary contusion appears as areas of airspace opacification that are usually in close proximity to the site of blunt trauma. Thus, the identification of consolidation adjacent to sites of rib fractures or bullet fragments should suggest the diagnosis. The consolidation from contusion typically appears on radiographs within 6 hours of the time of injury, and it usually improves within 24 to 72 hours. The consolidation usually completely resolves within 1 week of onset.

Pulmonary laceration refers to a tear in the lung parenchyma. Such injuries may initially be masked by surrounding contusion. On radiographs of patients with pulmonary laceration injury, you may observe an ovoid cystic lucency that represents a posttraumatic pneumatocele. Such cysts are typically small (5 mm to 1 cm), but larger cysts can be seen in some cases. If the cyst fills with blood, a spherical hematoma is observed. In some cases, the cyst contains air and blood, with a resultant air-fluid level.

Notes

Pneumomediastinum

1. Pneumomediastinum.

2. Yes—small apical pneumothoraces.

3. Alveolar rupture.

4. No.

Reference

Bejvan SM, Godwin JD: Pneumomediastinum: old signs and new signs. *AJR Am J Roentgenol* 166:1041–1048, 1996.

Cross-Reference

Thoracic Radiology: THE REQUISITES, p 172.

Comment

There are a variety of causes of pneumomediastinum. Intrathoracic sources include ruptured alveoli, tracheal perforation, and esophageal rupture. Air may also enter the mediastinum from the neck or retroperitoneum.

Alveolar rupture is the most common mechanism of pneumomediastinum and may occur secondary to elevated intraalveolar pressure or damage to alveolar walls. Causes of elevated intraalveolar pressure include airway obstruction (e.g., asthma, foreign body), mechanical ventilation, blunt thoracic trauma (the cause in this case), coughing, Valsalva maneuver, and vomiting. Disorders associated with alveolar wall damage include pneumonia, adult respiratory distress syndrome, emphysema, and interstitial fibrosis.

On radiographs of patients with pneumomediastinum, you will observe lucent streaks of air that surround the mediastinal structures, elevate the mediastinal pleura, and frequently extend into the soft tissues of the neck. In most cases, pneumomediastinum is readily distinguishable from pneumothorax and pneumopericardium. However, when only a small amount of gas is localized adjacent to the heart border, it may be difficult to distinguish these entities. In such cases, a lateral decubitus view may be helpful: unlike pneumothorax and pneumopericardium, pneumomediastinum will not shift in position.

Notes

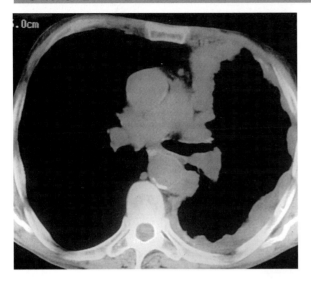
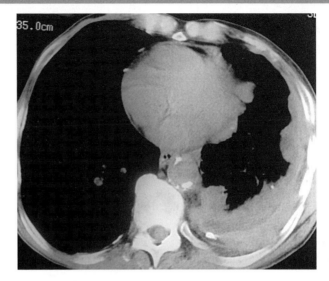

1. Name four features that are typical of malignant pleural thickening.

2. Which is more common: pleural metastases or malignant mesothelioma?

3. How frequently are pleural calcifications observed on CT scans of patients with malignant mesothelioma?

4. What is the typical latency period between exposure to asbestos and development of malignant mesothelioma?

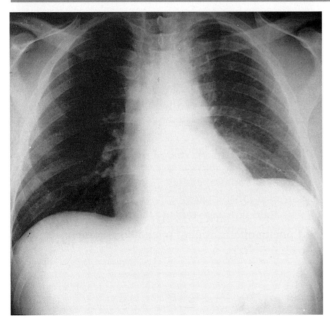
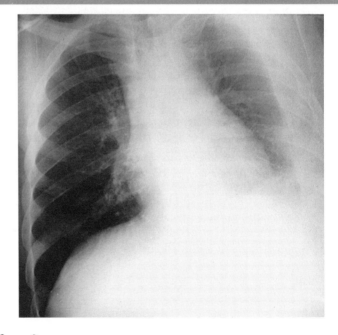

1. Where is the pleural effusion located in the first figure?

2. What is the most sensitive radiographic projection for detecting a pleural effusion?

3. How much pleural fluid must be present in order to observe blunting of the costophrenic angle on the frontal chest radiograph?

4. Name three causes of an exudative pleural effusion.

C A S E 1 5

Malignant Mesothelioma

1. More than 1 cm thick, circumferential, involves the mediastinal surface, and nodular.

2. Metastases.

3. Approximately 20%.

4. Between 30 and 40 years.

Reference

Miller BH, Rosado-de-Christenson ML, Mason AC, et al: Malignant pleural mesothelioma: radiologic-pathologic correlation. Radiographics 16:613–644, 1996.

Cross-Reference

Thoracic Radiology: THE REQUISITES, pp 505–511.

Comment

Malignant mesothelioma is the most common primary neoplasm of the pleura, but it is a relatively rare entity. In approximately 80% of cases, it affects individuals who have been exposed to asbestos. Males are affected more commonly than females. Presenting symptoms include chest pain and dyspnea.

The most common radiologic finding is the presence of diffuse pleural thickening, which is typically nodular and irregular in configuration. Diffuse pleural thickening is often accompanied by a reduction in the size of the affected hemithorax, with associated ipsilateral shift of the mediastinum. A pleural effusion is often present.

CT and MR are superior to radiography in assessing the extent of disease. In many cases, CT and MR play complementary roles in determining resectability. In particular, it is important to assess for transdiaphragmatic extension, diffuse chest wall invasion, invasion of vital mediastinal structures, vertebral body invasion, direct extension of tumor to the contralateral pleura, and distant metastases. The presence of one or more of these findings precludes surgical resection.

Patients with limited disease may be considered candidates for attempted surgical cure with an extrapleural pneumonectomy procedure. Regardless of therapy, however, malignant mesothelioma is almost always fatal.

Notes

C A S E 1 6

Subpulmonic Pleural Effusion

1. Subpulmonic space.

2. Lateral decubitus view.

3. At least 200 ml.

4. Infection, infarction, and neoplasm.

Reference

Kuhlman JE, Singha NK: Complex disease of the pleural space: radiologic and CT evaluation. *Radiographics* 17:63–79, 1997.

Cross-Reference

Thoracic Radiology: THE REQUISITES, pp 484–485.

Comment

On an upright chest radiograph, a pleural effusion is usually manifested by the presence of a "meniscus sign," which refers to a blunted appearance of the costophrenic angle, with a concave upward slope. In general, it requires approximately 200 ml of fluid to blunt the lateral costophrenic angle but only approximately 75 ml of fluid to blunt the posterior costophrenic angle. A lateral decubitus view can demonstrate as little as 5 ml of fluid.

In some patients, a large amount of free-flowing pleural fluid may collect in the subpulmonic space before spilling into the costophrenic angle. In such cases, you may observe a characteristic appearance on the frontal chest radiograph, including an apparent elevation of the hemidiaphragm, flattening of the diaphragm contour medially, and displacement of the peak of the diaphragm laterally. A suspected subpulmonic effusion can be confirmed by obtaining a lateral decubitus radiograph (second figure).

On the basis of laboratory evaluation, pleural effusions can be classified as exudates or transudates. Causes of exudates include infection, infarction, neoplasm, and inflammatory disorders. Causes of transudates include congestive heart failure, low protein level, myxedema, cirrhosis, nephrotic syndrome, and constrictive pericarditis.

Notes

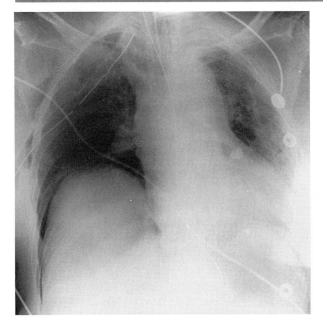

1. What abnormal extraalveolar intrathoracic air collection is evident on this supine chest radiograph?

2. What are the two most common locations of a pneumothorax on a supine radiograph?

3. On a supine radiograph, is an apicolateral visceral pleural line a highly sensitive sign for the diagnosis of pneumothorax?

4. Name at least three radiographic findings associated with a subpulmonic pneumothorax on a supine radiograph.

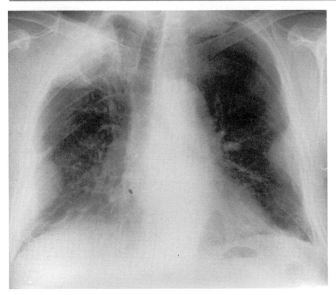

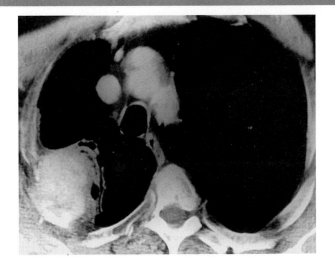

1. Where are these masses located?

2. Which feature is most helpful for differentiating a pleural mass from an extrapleural (chest wall) mass?

3. What are the two most common causes of an extrapleural mass with associated rib destruction in an adult patient?

4. Name two causes of hypervascular chest wall metastases.

Pneumothorax on Supine Radiograph

1. Pneumothorax.

2. Anteromedial and subpulmonic.

3. No.

4. Hyperlucent upper abdominal quadrant, deep sulcus sign, sharp diaphragmatic contour, and double diaphragm sign (this sign refers to visualization of the anterior and posterior surfaces of the diaphragm).

Reference

Tocino I, Westcott JL: Barotrauma. *Radiol Clin North Am* 34:59–81, 1996.

Cross-Reference

Thoracic Radiology: THE REQUISITES, p 170.

Comment

A pneumothorax is usually readily identifiable on an upright chest radiograph as an apicolateral white line (the visceral pleural line) with an absence of vessels beyond it. However, in the supine position, the apicolateral portion of the lung is no longer the most nondependent portion. Rather, air collects preferentially in the anteromedial and subpulmonic portions of the chest. Only when a very large volume of air is present in the pleural space will you visualize an apicolateral pleural line on a supine radiograph. Thus, although highly specific for pneumothorax, this is not a highly sensitive sign on supine radiographs.

The chest radiograph in this case shows several signs associated with a subpulmonic pneumothorax, including a hyperlucent appearance of the right upper quadrant of the abdomen, a deep costophrenic sulcus, and a sharp right hemidiaphragm contour. Also note the sharp outline of the right cardiac and mediastinal contours, findings associated with anteromedial pneumothorax.

Notes

Extrapleural Masses Secondary to Metastatic Thyroid Carcinoma

1. Extrapleural (chest wall).

2. The presence of rib abnormalities such as destruction or remodeling suggests an extrapleural location.

3. Metastatic disease and myeloma.

4. Thyroid carcinoma and renal cell carcinoma.

Reference

Reed JC: Chest wall lesions. In: *Chest Radiology: Plain Film Patterns and Differential Diagnoses*, fourth edition. St. Louis, Mosby–Year Book, 1997, pp 6–21.

Cross-Reference

Thoracic Radiology: THE REQUISITES, pp 48–49.

Comment

The chest radiograph shows multiple masses that form obtuse angles with the adjacent chest wall and have incomplete, tapered borders. Such an appearance is typical of an intrathoracic, extrapulmonary location. The identification of rib destruction (best seen on the CT image) confirms that the masses are extrapleural.

In an adult patient, the most common causes of chest wall masses with associated rib destruction are metastatic disease and multiple myeloma. The contrast-enhanced CT image shows intense enhancement of the mass, a finding that is associated with hypervascular metastases. The most common causes for such findings are metastatic thyroid carcinoma and renal cell carcinoma.

Notes

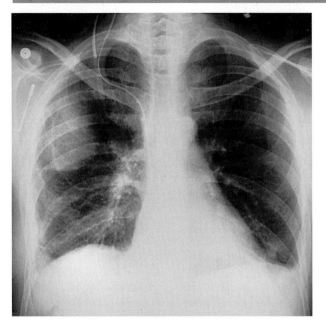 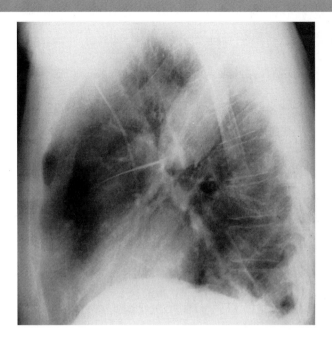

1. What is the location of the confluent opacity in the right lung?

2. What feature of this opacity on the PA projection suggests an extraparenchymal location?

3. What features of this opacity suggest a pleural location on the lateral projection?

4. What is the term used to describe a mass-like opacity due to loculated pleural fluid within a fissure?

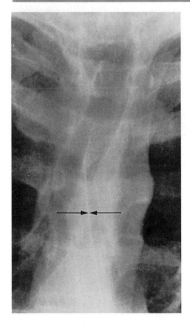

1. Name the mediastinal line that is demonstrated (arrows).

2. How many layers of pleura form this line?

3. Which line extends above the level of the clavicles—the anterior or the posterior junction line?

4. Which line is visualized more frequently—the anterior or the posterior junction line?

Loculated Pleural Fluid in the Major Fissure

1. Pleura (the major fissure).

2. Incomplete borders (note the sharp margins inferomedially and the lack of a distinct margin superolaterally).

3. Elliptical configuration and an oblique orientation corresponding to the course of the major fissure.

4. Vanishing tumor, phantom tumor, or pseudotumor.

Reference

Wilson AG: Pleura and pleural disorders. In: Armstrong P, Wilson AG, Dee P, Hansell DM, Eds: *Imaging of Diseases of the Chest*, second edition. St. Louis, Mosby, 1995, pp 661–667.

Cross-Reference

Thoracic Radiology: THE REQUISITES, p 485.

Comment

The chest radiograph in this case demonstrates the characteristic appearance of a loculated pleural fluid collection within the major fissure. Such loculation occurs most commonly in patients with heart failure. Loculated fluid is seen more often in the right lung than the left, and the minor fissure is more commonly involved than the major fissure. Because of the transient nature of loculated fluid collections, they have been referred to as "vanishing tumors," "phantom tumors," and "pseudotumors." Such terms should be avoided in radiology reports to avoid possible confusion.

When fluid is loculated within the major fissure, it may appear on the PA projection as either a discrete, mass-like opacity with incomplete borders (as demonstrated in the first figure) or as a hazy, veil-like opacity. On the lateral radiograph, such a loculated fluid collection appears as a well-marginated, elliptical opacity coursing along the obliquely oriented axis of the major fissure (as demonstrated in the second figure). The rapid onset and resolution of such fluid collections usually allow one to readily distinguish loculated fluid from a solid pleural mass. When the diagnosis is in doubt, a decubitus view may be helpful, because it will demonstrate the free fluid to shift in distribution.

Notes

Anterior Junction Line

1. Anterior junction line.

2. Four.

3. Posterior junction line.

4. Anterior junction line.

Reference

Fraser RS, Müller NL, Colman N, Paré PD: The mediastinum. In: *Fraser and Paré's Diagnosis of Disease of the Chest,* fourth edition. Philadelphia, WB Saunders, 1999, pp 201–204.

Cross-Reference

Thoracic Radiology: THE REQUISITES, pp 421–423.

Comment

The coned-down frontal radiograph demonstrates the normal appearance of the anterior junction line, which is formed by the close apposition of the visceral and parietal layers of pleura of both lungs as they approximate anterior to the mediastinum. Similarly, the posterior junction line (not visible in this case) represents the apposition of pleural layers of both lungs as they approximate posterior to the mediastinum.

The anterior portion of the thorax begins at the thoracic inlet. Thus, the anterior junction line begins at the undersurface of the clavicles. It typically courses obliquely from right to left, as demonstrated in this case. The posterior portion of the thorax extends more superiorly than the anterior portion. Thus, the posterior junction line may be seen above the level of the clavicles. In contrast with the anterior junction line, it typically appears as a straight vertical line, often visible through the tracheal air column.

The identification of a displaced junction line can help you identify and localize a mediastinal mass. Displacement of a junction line is also an indicator of volume loss and may accompany atelectasis of a lobe or lung.

Notes

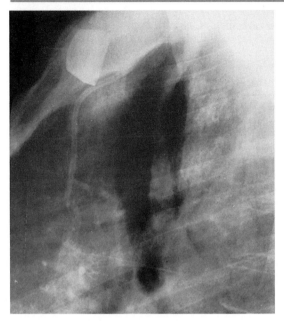
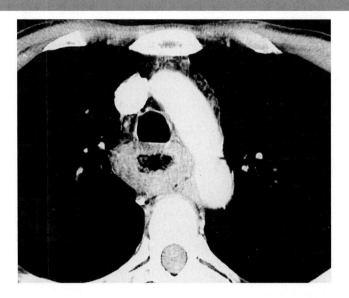

1. What is the most likely cause of the thickened tracheoesophageal stripe observed on the lateral chest radiograph?
2. What are the major risk factors for developing esophageal carcinoma?
3. What is the most common cell type of esophageal neoplasm?
4. What is the most common benign esophageal neoplasm?

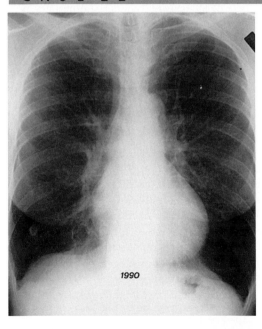
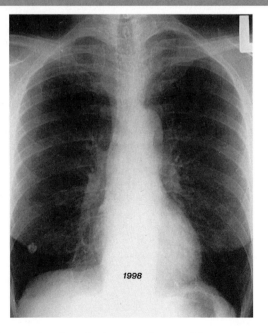

1. Measurements of this nodule show no change in size during the interval between these two radiographs. Is this nodule benign, indeterminate, or malignant?
2. Name at least three benign calcification patterns.
3. Name at least one calcification pattern that is not considered benign.
4. Are follow-up radiographs or CT necessary to further evaluate this nodule?

Esophageal Carcinoma

1. Esophageal carcinoma.

2. Cigarette smoking and alcohol ingestion (additional risk factors include achalasia, preexisting benign stricture, Barrett's esophagus, tylosis, Plummer-Vinson syndrome, and sprue).

3. Squamous cell carcinoma.

4. Leiomyoma.

Reference

Fraser RS, Müller NL, Colman N, Paré PD: The mediastinum. In: *Fraser and Paré's Diagnosis of Diseases of the Chest*, fourth edition. Philadelphia, WB Saunders, 1999, pp 221-223.

Cross-Reference

Thoracic Radiology: THE REQUISITES, pp 455-457.

Comment

The lateral chest radiograph demonstrates abnormal thickening of the tracheoesophageal stripe and anterior displacement of the trachea. A tracheoesophageal stripe that measures more than 5 mm in width should be considered abnormal and usually signifies the presence of esophageal carcinoma. The CT image confirms the presence of esophageal wall thickening. Images below this level (not shown) demonstrated an obstructing esophageal neoplasm.

In patients with esophageal carcinoma, CT can be helpful for assessing the extent of the primary esophageal lesion, identifying nodal spread, and determining extension of the neoplasm beyond the esophagus. CT is often used in conjunction with other modalities such as endoscopy and endoscopic ultrasonography for staging purposes.

Notes

Benign Calcified Granuloma

1. Benign.

2. Diffuse, central, popcorn, and laminar (concentric).

3. Eccentric; stippled.

4. No.

References

Erasmus JJ, Connoly JE, McAdams HP, Roggli VL: Solitary pulmonary nodules: part I. Morphologic evaluation for differentiation of benign and malignant lesions. *Radiographics*, 20:43-58, 2000.

Erasmus JJ, McAdams HP, Connoly JE: Solitary pulmonary nodules: part II. Evaluation of the indeterminate nodule. *Radiographics* 20:59-66, 2000.

Cross-Reference

Thoracic Radiology: THE REQUISITES, pp 340-343.

Comment

The chest radiographs demonstrate stability in size of a small right lower lobe nodule over an 8-year period. Note the presence of laminar calcification, a recognized benign pattern.

There are two accepted radiographic criteria for a benign solitary pulmonary nodule: (1) lack of interval growth for at least 2 years and (2) identification of a benign calcification pattern within a smoothly marginated pulmonary nodule.

Roughly half of all resected solitary pulmonary nodules prove to be benign. Clinical indicators that suggest a benign diagnosis include age younger than 35 years and history of exposure to tuberculosis or residence in an endemic granuloma area. Such indicators are, unfortunately, insufficiently specific to be helpful in most individual cases.

For patients with nodules that do not meet the accepted radiographic criteria for benignancy, non-contrast CT with thin-section imaging is usually the preferred method for further evaluation. CT is more sensitive than conventional radiographs for detecting calcium and fat within a nodule. In certain cases, CT imaging allows a confident diagnosis of a specific benign entity such as granuloma, hamartoma, arteriovenous malformation, pulmonary infarction, mucoid impaction, and pulmonary sequestration.

When CT is nondiagnostic, the method of further evaluation depends on patient characteristics and nodule morphology. Noninvasive imaging modalities include contrast-enhanced CT to assess for abnormal nodule enhancement and 2-[fluorine-18] fluoro-2-deoxy-D-glucose (FDG) positron emission tomography (PET) imaging, which relies on abnormal glucose analog (FDG) uptake to distinguish benign from malignant nodules.

Notes

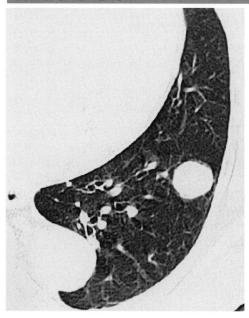
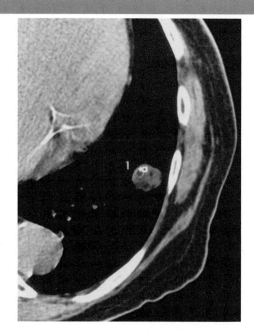

1. CT density measurements of this nodule revealed areas of low attenuation, measuring approximately −60 Hounsfield units. What type of tissue is associated with this Hounsfield measurement?
2. What is the diagnosis for this solitary pulmonary nodule?
3. Is this a benign or a malignant entity?
4. Are hamartomas always stable in size over time?

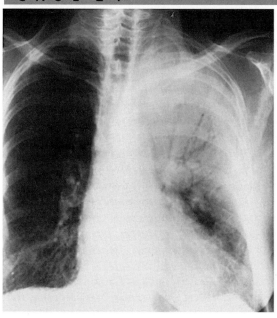
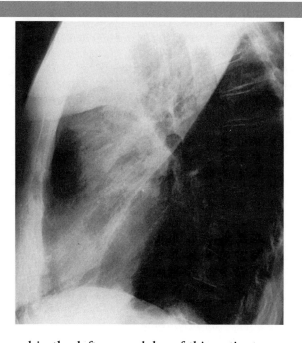

1. Name the pattern of lung opacification observed in the left upper lobe of this patient.
2. What is the term used to describe the air-filled, tubular, branching structures that are visible within the left upper lobe?
3. Name at least three substances that may fill the alveolar spaces and produce an alveolar consolidation pattern.
4. Name the organism that is most frequently associated with lobar pneumonia in the normal (nonimmunosuppressed) host.

C A S E   2 3

Hamartoma

1. Fat.

2. Hamartoma.

3. Benign.

4. No.

Reference
Siegelman SS, Khori NF, Scott WW, et al: Pulmonary hamartoma: CT findings. *Radiology* 160:313-317, 1986.

Cross-Reference
Thoracic Radiology: THE REQUISITES, pp 302-304.

Comment
The thin-section CT images demonstrate a well-circumscribed, spherical, solitary pulmonary nodule within the periphery of the left lower lobe. The nodule contains several low attenuation areas, which represent focal deposits of fat. The identification of fat deposits (-50 to -150 Hounsfield units) within a pulmonary nodule is diagnostic of a hamartoma, the most common benign pulmonary neoplasm.

A hamartoma is an acquired lesion that represents a disorganized growth of tissue normally found within the lung. Pathologically, the tumors contain cartilage, fibrous tissue, and mature fat cells. Other mesenchymal elements such as bone, vessels, and smooth muscle may also be present.

Affected patients range in age from 30 to 70 years, with a peak incidence observed in the sixth decade of life. There is a slight female predominance. The majority of lesions are detected incidentally on routine chest radiographs of asymptomatic patients. An exception is the presence of an endobronchial hamartoma, which may present with symptoms of airway obstruction.

On imaging studies, hamartomas typically appear as well-defined, solitary, spherical nodules or masses. A characteristic "popcorn" pattern of calcification is identified in approximately 10% to 15% of cases on conventional radiographs and in approximately 25% of cases on CT imaging. Hamartomas typically grow slowly and may rarely be multiple.

Thin-section CT evaluation is more accurate than conventional radiography for diagnosing hamartoma. In the majority of cases, CT will demonstrate one of the following patterns: focal or diffuse fat attenuation; a combination of fat and calcification; or diffuse popcorn calcification.

Notes

C A S E   2 4

Left Upper Lobe Pneumonia

1. Alveolar consolidation.

2. Air bronchograms.

3. Water (edema), pus (pneumonia), blood (hemorrhage), cells (bronchioalveolar cell carcinoma), and protein (alveolar proteinosis).

4. *Streptococcus pneumoniae.*

Reference
Armstrong P, Dee P: Infections of the lungs and pleura. In: Armstrong P, Wilson AG, Dee P, Hansell DM, Eds: *Imaging of Diseases of the Chest*, second edition. St. Louis, Mosby, 1995, pp 145-149.

Cross-Reference
Thoracic Radiology: THE REQUISITES, pp 31-33, 92-95.

Comment
The chest radiograph demonstrates the presence of confluent opacification within the left upper lobe with prominent air bronchograms, consistent with alveolar consolidation. This pattern may be caused by the accumulation of edema, pus, hemorrhage, cells, or protein within the alveolar spaces.

Once you have identified a pattern of alveolar consolidation, it is important to determine the distribution and chronicity of the process. You should also correlate the imaging findings with the clinical presentation of the patient.

The distribution of alveolar consolidation is often quite helpful in narrowing the differential diagnosis. For example, the presence of a bilateral, perihilar distribution of alveolar consolidation is most suggestive of hydrostatic pulmonary edema. In contrast, this case demonstrates a striking lobar distribution of consolidation, a pattern that is most commonly associated with pneumonia. The most common organism to produce a lobar pneumonia is *S. pneumoniae*. Other organisms such as *Klebsiella pneumoniae*, *Legionella pneumophila*, and *Mycoplasma pneumoniae* may also produce a lobar consolidation pattern.

With regard to the chronicity of a consolidative pattern, this factor is best determined by comparing the current study with prior chest radiographs. The presence of chronic consolidation is associated with a limited differential diagnosis that includes bronchoalveolar cell carcinoma, alveolar proteinosis, lipoid pneumonia, lymphoma, and the "alveolar" form of sarcoid.

Notes

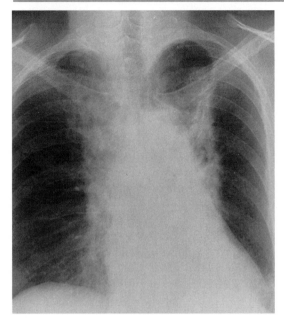

1. In this patient with a history of Hodgkin's lymphoma, what is the most likely etiology of the paramediastinal lung parenchymal opacification?

2. Is this a common finding in patients who have received mantle radiation therapy for lymphoma?

3. At what time point following completion of radiation therapy is radiation pneumonitis usually detectable by chest radiography?

4. Name the term that is used to describe the presence of dilated bronchi within areas of fibrosis.

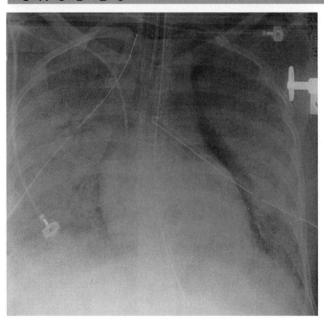

1. Define the adult respiratory distress syndrome (ARDS).

2. Name at least three common causes.

3. What sign of barotrauma is evident in this patient?

4. What is the distribution of this abnormal, extraalveolar air collection?

CASE 25

Radiation Pneumonitis

1. Radiation pneumonitis.

2. Yes.

3. Approximately 6 to 8 weeks.

4. Traction bronchiectasis.

Reference

Dee P: Drug- and radiation-induced lung disease. In: Armstrong P, Wilson AG, Dee P, Hansell DM, Eds: *Imaging of Diseases of the Chest*, second edition. St. Louis, Mosby, pp 477–482.

Cross-Reference

Thoracic Radiology: THE REQUISITES, pp 331–334.

Comment

The chest radiograph demonstrates a bilateral, paramediastinal distribution of parenchymal opacification with associated air bronchograms. The geographic margins and geometric shape correspond to the field of irradiation.

Radiation pneumonitis and fibrosis are observed in the majority of patients who have received mantle radiation therapy for lymphoma. Radiation pneumonitis is generally observed on chest radiographs within 6 to 8 weeks following completion of treatment, but CT may detect subtle abnormalities earlier than radiography. Such opacities are characteristically sharply demarcated and are not limited by anatomic boundaries such as fissures. Fibrosis usually develops within 6 to 12 months following radiation therapy. With time, the parenchymal opacities generally become more linear in configuration and are usually accompanied by volume loss and traction bronchiectasis.

Notes

CASE 26

Adult Respiratory Distress Syndrome Complicated by Left Anteromedial Pneumothorax From Barotrauma

1. ARDS is a clinical diagnosis of acute respiratory failure characterized by profound hypoxia accompanied by diffuse parenchymal opacification on chest radiography.

2. Trauma, sepsis, severe pneumonia, circulatory shock, aspiration, inhaled toxins, drug overdose, and multiple transfusions.

3. Pneumothorax.

4. Anteromedial.

Reference

Boiselle PM: Radiologic imaging in the critically ill patient. In: Criner GJ, D'Alonzo G, Eds: *Critical Care Manual*. New York, Springer-Verlag, in press.

Cross-Reference

Thoracic Radiology: THE REQUISITES, pp 169–172.

Comment

The chest radiograph of a patient who attempted suicide by drug overdose reveals diffuse bilateral lung opacification with prominent air bronchograms. Allowing for portable, supine technique, the heart does not appear enlarged. Note the prominent lucency along the left mediastinal contour, corresponding to an anteromedial left pneumothorax.

ARDS is a form of noncardiogenic pulmonary edema caused by increased capillary permeability. In contrast with patients with hydrostatic (cardiogenic) pulmonary edema, the heart size and vascular pedicle width of patients with ARDS are usually normal. Moreover, common features of hydrostatic edema such as pleural effusions, Kerley (septal) lines, and peribronchial cuffing are not usually evident in patients with ARDS. When the vessels are visible in patients with ARDS, they are often constricted. Finally, although both ARDS and hydrostatic edema are associated with airspace consolidation, the distribution often differs between these two entities. Early in the course of ARDS, the opacities are often patchy and somewhat peripheral in distribution. In contrast, patients with hydrostatic edema more often demonstrate confluent opacities with a central, perihilar predominance. Air bronchograms are visible more frequently in patients with ARDS than in those with hydrostatic edema. As ARDS progresses, areas of consolidation are frequently replaced by fibrosis and cyst formation.

Because of decreased lung compliance and the need for prolonged mechanical ventilation, patients with ARDS frequently develop barotrauma, including subcutaneous emphysema, pneumothorax, pneumomediastinum, and pulmonary interstitial emphysema.

Notes

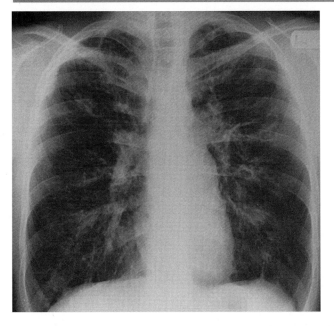
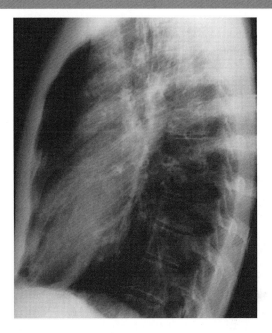

1. Name two radiographic signs of bronchiectasis that are present in this case.
2. What is the most likely cause of bronchiectasis that is most severe in the upper lobes?
3. How is this condition inherited?
4. Does this condtion ever initially present in adulthood?

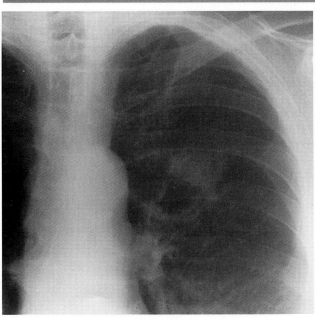
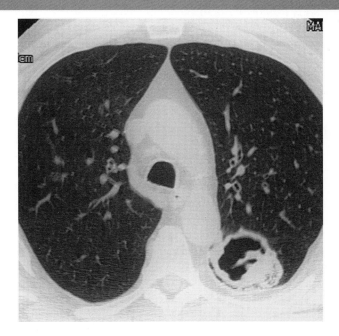

1. Can you reliably distinguish between an infectious and a neoplastic etiology of a cavity based on imaging features alone?
2. Based on the location of this cavity, what is the most important infectious consideration?
3. In addition to infectious and neoplastic causes, what other categories of abnormalities should you consider when a patient presents with one or more cavities?
4. Which cell type of lung cancer is most closely associated with the presence of cavitation?

Cystic Fibrosis

1. Bronchial wall thickening ("tram-tracking") and cysts ("ring shadows").

2. Cystic fibrosis (CF).

3. Autosomal recessive.

4. Yes—occasionally mild forms of CF are first diagnosed in adult patients.

Reference

Webb WR: Radiology of obstructive lung disease. *AJR Am J Roentgenol* 169:637-647, 1997.

Cross-Reference

Thoracic Radiology: THE REQUISITES, pp 391-394.

Comment

The chest radiographs in this case demonstrate cylindrical bronchiectasis, manifested by bronchial wall thickening (tram-tracking) and cysts (ring shadows). Although the distribution is diffuse, the bronchiectasis is most severe in the upper lobes. Also note the presence of tubular opacities, most pronounced in the right upper lobe, corresponding to foci of mucoid impaction. The lungs appear hyperinflated, with prominence of the retrosternal clear space. The findings are typical of CF, a hereditary disorder characterized by abnormal secretions from exocrine glands, including the airways, pancreas, large bowel, and salivary and sweat glands. The major clinical manifestations of this disorder are chronic pulmonary disease due to bronchiectasis and pancreatic insufficiency.

Although CF is usually diagnosed during infancy or childhood, milder forms of the disease are occasionally first diagnosed in adults. Affected patients are at increased risk for pulmonary infections with a variety of organisms, including *Staphylococcus aureus*, *Pseudomonas aeruginosa*, *Haemophilus influenzae*, and *Pseudomonas cepacia*. The last organism is a major cause of infection late in the course of CF. Presenting symptoms are related to recurrent pulmonary infections and include productive cough, wheezing, dyspnea, and hemoptysis. The diagnosis of CF may be confirmed by an abnormal sweat test or molecular biologic testing (polymerase chain reaction).

Classic chest radiograph findings include bronchial wall thickening, cystic spaces due to dilated airways, hyperinflation, and mucoid impaction. Recurrent foci of consolidation and atelectasis are commonly observed. Hilar enlargement is frequently seen in adult patients (note the enlarged hila in this case) and may occur secondary to hilar lymph node enlargement or pulmonary artery hypertension.

Notes

Cavity Due to Reactivation Tuberculosis

1. No.

2. Reactivation TB.

3. Vasculitis and granulomatoses.

4. Squamous cell carcinoma.

Reference

Reed JC: Solitary localized lucent defect. In: *Chest Radiology: Plain Film Patterns and Differential Diagnoses*, fourth edition. St. Louis, Mosby-Year Book, 1997, pp 390-411.

Cross-Reference

Thoracic Radiology: THE REQUISITES, pp 49-58.

Comment

The term *cavity* refers to a lucency located within a nodule, mass, or focus of consolidation. There are a variety of causes, including infection (pyogenic and granulomatous), neoplasm (usually squamous cell), vasculitides and granulomatoses, and, rarely, infarction. The most common causes of a solitary cavity are infections and neoplasms.

Certain features can help you determine the likely cause of a cavity, but they are not specific enough to allow you to make a definitive diagnosis in most cases. Features to consider include wall thickness, presence or absence of a fluid level, location, and presence of adjacent lung parenchymal abnormalities. With regard to wall thickness, very thin-walled (<4-mm-diameter) cavities are often benign. In contrast, neoplasms typically demonstrate very thick walls. There is considerable overlap in this feature, however, and it should not be used as a sole criterion. With regard to the presence of a fluid level, it is most often associated with benign nodules; however, fluid levels may occasionally be observed in cavitary neoplasms that have been complicated by secondary infection or hemorrhage. Regarding the location of a cavity, hematogenous cavities often have a lower lobe predominance, reflecting the gravitational distribution of blood flow. Cavities associated with reactivation TB are most commonly located in the apical and posterior segments of the upper lobes and the superior segments of the lower lobes. Primary lung cancer is most common in the upper lobes, but any lobe may be affected. Regarding the presence of adjacent lung abnormalities, the development of a cavity within a preexisting area of consolidation is typical of a lung abscess.

Notes

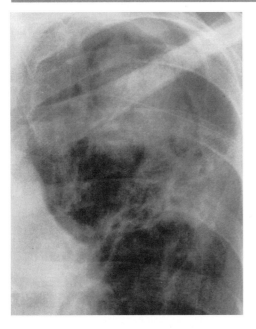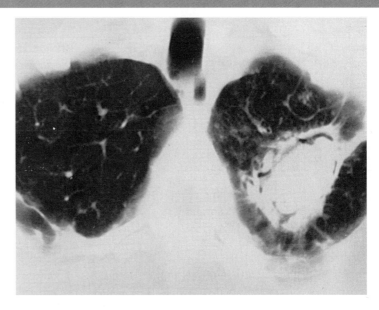

1. What is the most likely cause for this intracavitary mass?
2. What pleural abnormality frequently accompanies the development of a mycetoma?
3. What is the usual treatment for asymptomatic individuals with this finding?
4. Name at least two therapeutic options for patients who develop hemoptysis from this process.

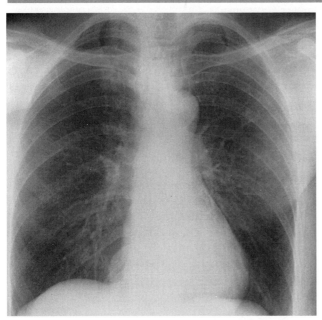

1. Name at least four possible causes for a right cardiophrenic angle mass.
2. Which one of these entities is characterized by fluid contents?
3. Are pericardial cysts more common on the right or the left side?
4. Do pericardial cysts usually communicate with the pericardium?

Mycetoma

1. Mycetoma.

2. Pleural thickening.

3. None.

4. Bronchial artery embolization, direct instillation of amphotericin B via a percutaneous catheter into the cavity, and surgical resection.

Reference

Thompson BH, Stanford W, Galvin JR, Kurihara Y: Varied radiologic appearances of pulmonary aspergillosis. *Radiographics* 15:1273-1284, 1995.

Cross-Reference

Thoracic Radiology: THE REQUISITES, pp 128-129.

Comment

The chest radiograph and chest CT images demonstrate the presence of an intracavitary left upper lobe mass and apical pleural thickening. The imaging findings are characteristic of an aspergilloma, the most common radiographic form of aspergillosis.

Aspergilloma (also called *mycetoma*) refers to a saprophytic infection that occurs within a preexisting cyst, cavity, bulla, or area of bronchiectasis. Pathologically, the fungus ball is shown to represent a combination of *Aspergillus* hyphae, mucus, and cellular debris.

Patients at risk for aspergilloma formation include those with CF, sarcoidosis, TB, and emphysema. The infection is typically clinically silent for many years. Presenting symptoms may include cough, weight loss, and recurrent hemoptysis. Although hemoptysis is usually minimal, a minority of patients may present with massive, life-threatening hemoptysis. Severe hemoptysis requires therapeutic intervention such as bronchial artery embolization.

Characteristic imaging findings include a round, dependent opacity located within a cavity or thin-walled cyst. The dependent opacity is often heterogeneous due to the presence of multiple linear collections of air, resulting in a "sponge-like" appearance. It occurs most commonly in the upper lobes and is frequently accompanied by pleural thickening. In a majority of cases, the fungus ball demonstrates mobility on changes in patient positioning. An aspergilloma is often surrounded by a crescent of air, referred to as the "monad sign." In a minority of cases, however, the fungus ball may completely fill the cavity, with no visible air between the cavity and the ball.

Notes

Pericardial Cyst

1. Pericardial fat pad, pericardial cyst, Morgagni's foramen hernia, lipoma, thymolipoma, and enlarged epicardial lymph nodes.

2. Pericardial cyst.

3. Right side.

4. No.

Reference

Armstrong P: Mediastinal and hilar disorders. In: Armstrong P, Wilson AG, Dee P, Hansell DM, Eds: *Imaging of Diseases of the Chest*, second edition. St. Louis, Mosby, 1995, pp 736-738.

Cross-Reference

Thoracic Radiology: THE REQUISITES, pp 449-452.

Comment

The chest radiograph demonstrates a well-marginated right cardiophrenic angle mass. The majority of causes of a right cardiophrenic angle mass are benign, as listed in Answer 1.

Although the various causes of a right cardiophrenic angle mass may appear similar radiographically, the CT appearances differ depending on the contents of the lesion. The presence of fluid attenuation within a cardiophrenic angle mass is consistent with a pericardial cyst, the diagnosis in this case. Such cysts are attached to the parietal pericardium, but they do not usually communicate with the pericardial space.

The presence of fat attenuation within a cardiophrenic angle mass can be seen in lipoma, thymolipoma, and Morgagni's foramen hernia. Lipomas usually demonstrate homogeneous fat attenuation. Thymolipomas, on the other hand, contain a variable mixture of fat and soft tissue elements. Herniated omental fat can be distinguished by the identification of omental vessels, which appear as serpiginous, tubular soft tissue densities. In many cases, herniated omental fat is also accompanied by bowel and/or liver. Occasionally, herniated bowel is visible radiographically, allowing you to make a specific diagnosis of this entity.

A soft tissue attenuation cardiophrenic angle mass is suggestive of enlarged epicardial lymph nodes. Such nodes are a common site of recurrence in patients with Hodgkin's disease.

Notes

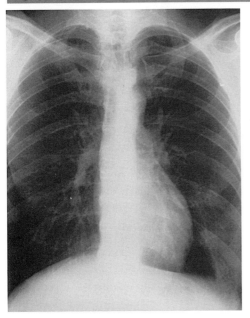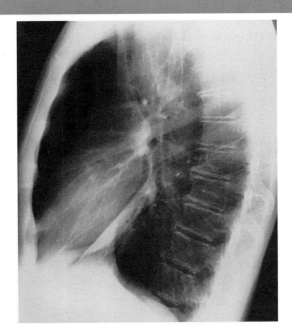

1. In which segment of the lung is the consolidation located?
2. What numbered bronchopulmonary segments does this correspond to?
3. Name the order of left lower lobe basilar segmental bronchi from lateral to medial on a frontal radiograph.
4. What is the order on the right side?

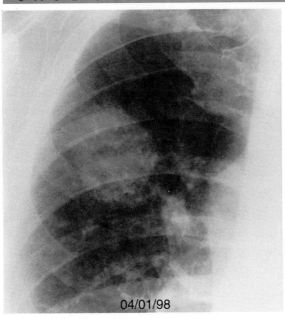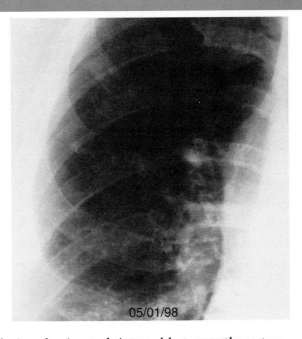

04/01/98   05/01/98

1. This patient received a course of antibiotics during the 1-month interval between these two radiographs (the first figure preceded the second). What is the likely diagnosis?
2. What organism is most closely associated with a round pneumonia?
3. Are round pneumonias more common in adult or pediatric patients?
4. Based only on the findings in the first figure, what is the most important differential diagnosis to consider?

C A S E   3 1

Pneumonia of the Anteromedial Basal Segment of the Left Lower Lobe

1. Anteromedial segment of the left lower lobe.

2. Segments 7 and 8.

3. Anteromedial, lateral, and posterior (ALP).

4. Anterior, lateral, posterior, and medial.

Reference

Freundlich IM: Anatomy. In: Freundlich IM, Bragg DG, Eds: *A Radiologic Approach to Diseases of the Chest*, Baltimore, Williams & Wilkins, 1992, pp 29-43.

Cross-Reference

Thoracic Radiology: THE REQUISITES, pp 7-10.

Comment

The frontal radiograph in the first figure demonstrates a subtle focus of parenchymal opacification in the left lower lobe laterally. The focal consolidation is seen in better detail on the lateral radiograph, where it is sharply marginated anteriorly by the major fissure. This location corresponds anatomically to the anteromedial segment of the left lower lobe.

Note the characteristic lateral location of the anteromedial segment on the frontal chest radiograph. The order of the left lower lobe basilar segments on the frontal radiograph (from lateral to medial) is anteromedial, lateral, and posterior (ALP). In the right lower lobe, the order of the basilar segments (from lateral to medial) is anterior, lateral, posterior, and medial.

Notes

C A S E   3 2

Round Pneumonia

1. Round pneumonia.

2. *Streptococcus pneumoniae*.

3. Pediatric.

4. Bronchogenic carcinoma.

Reference

Wagner AL, Szabunio M, Hazlett KS, Wagner SG: Radiologic manifestations of round pneumonia in adults. *AJR Am J Roentgenol*, 170:723-726, 1998.

Cross-Reference

Thoracic Radiology: THE REQUISITES, pp 101-102.

Comment

Pneumonia may occasionally manifest as a rounded, mass-like opacity with either smooth or irregular margins. Round pneumonia is seen much more frequentlly in children than adults and is most commonly associated with pneumococcal pneumonia.

When an adult patient presents with a rounded, mass-like opacity, bronchogenic carcinoma is the most important diagnosis to consider. Because neoplasms (especially bronchoalveolar cell carcinoma and lymphoma) may occasionally be associated with air bronchograms, the presence or absence of this finding is not helpful in distinguishing infection from neoplasm. Moreover, only a minority of cases of round pneumonia demonstrate air bronchograms radiographically.

A recent chest radiograph with normal findings and a history of infectious symptoms can aid in the diagnosis of round pneumonia. In adult patients with a suspected diagnosis of round pneumonia, follow-up radiographs following appropriate antibiotic therapy are mandatory. Failure of a rounded opacity to completely resolve following antibiotic therapy generally warrants further evaluation with invasive procedures to exclude neoplasm.

Notes

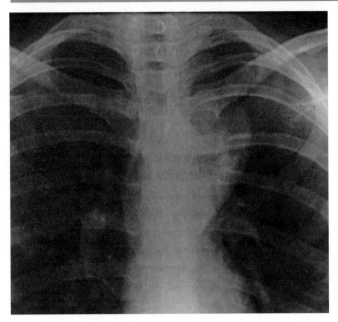

1. Name two features of this mass that are suggestive of a mediastinal location.
2. What osseous abnormality is associated with this mass?
3. Does this osseous finding imply a malignant etiology?
4. What is the most common cause of a posterior mediastinal mass?

Neurogenic Tumor (Ganglioneuroma)

1. Smooth, sharp margins and obtuse angle with the adjacent lung.

2. Rib spreading (left fourth and fifth posterior ribs).

3. No.

4. Neurogenic tumor.

Reference

Strollo DC, Rosado-de-Christenson ML, Jett JR: Primary mediastinal tumors: part II. Tumors of the middle and posterior mediastinum. *Chest* 112:1344–1357, 1997.

Cross-Reference

Thoracic Radiology: THE REQUISITES, pp 427–429, 452–453.

Comment

Neurogenic tumors are the most common cause of a posterior mediastinal mass. Such lesions can be classified into three groups: (1) those arising from peripheral nerves (schwannoma, neurofibroma); (2) those arising from the sympathetic chain (ganglioneuroma, ganglioneuroblastoma, neuroblastoma); and (3) those arising from the paraganglia (pheochromocytoma, chemodectoma). The majority of lesions (roughly 70%) are benign.

Neurogenic tumors typically affect patients during the first 4 decades of life. Most lesions are detected incidentally in asymptomatic patients. Symptomatic lesions typically produce neurologic symptoms such as radicular pain and neuresthesias. Intravertebral extension may result in symptoms of cord compression.

Interestingly, tumors arising from peripheral nerves, such as schwannoma, tend to differ in shape from those arising from the sympathetic chain, such as ganglioneuroma. The former lesions are generally round and the latter are usually fusiform, with a vertical orientation. Note the fusiform shape and vertical orientation of the mass in this case, which is typical of a ganglioneuroma.

Rib abnormalities such as rib spreading and rib erosion are commonly associated with neurogenic tumors and do not imply malignancy. In contrast, the presence of bone destruction is suspicious for malignancy. Vertebral body abnormalities are commonly present. Such abnormalities are best demonstrated on CT examinations. Tumors arising from peripheral nerves are often associated with widening of the neural foramen. In contrast, those lesions arising from the sympathetic chain more often result in anterolateral vertebral body erosion.

On cross-sectional imaging studies, benign neurogenic tumors are usually homogeneous in appearance and have well-defined margins. Malignant lesions are more likely to appear heterogeneous and to demonstrate irregular margins.

Foci of calcification are present in a minority of cases. Such calcifications are more often identified on CT than on chest radiographs. Note the presence of focal calcification on the chest radiograph in this case. Calcification is more commonly observed in tumors arising from the sympathetic chain than in those arising from the peripheral nerves.

Once you have identified a suspected neurogenic tumor on chest radiographs, MRI is generally the preferred cross-sectional imaging modality for further evaluation because of its superb ability to demonstrate intraspinal extension of tumor or the presence of an associated spinal cord abnormality.

Notes

Fair Game

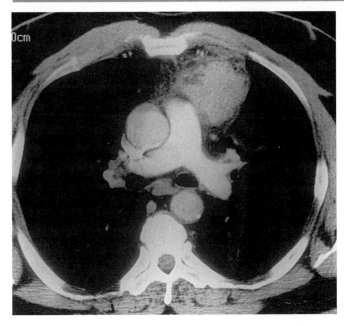

1. In what mediastinal compartment is this mass located?
2. The majority of anterior mediastinal masses in adult patients arise in which organ?
3. Name at least three causes of thymic masses.
4. How do the metastatic patterns of invasive thymoma and thymic carcinoma differ?

↓ Azygoesophageal interface

C A S E   3 5

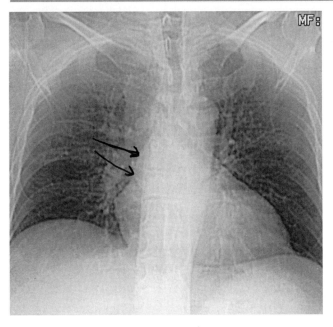 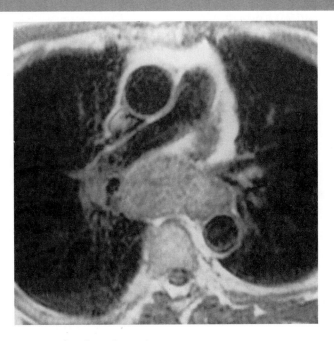

1. What is the differential diagnosis for the subcarinal mass in the first figure?
2. Based on the MRI, what is the most likely diagnosis?
3. Name at least three sites of primary neoplasms that commonly result in metastatic intrathoracic lymphadenopathy.
4. What mediastinal interface is displaced laterally in the first figure?

Thymic Mass (Thymic Carcinoma)

1. Anterior.

2. Thymus.

3. Thymoma, thymic hyperplasia, thymolipoma, thymic cyst, thymic carcinoma, and thymic carcinoid.

4. Only thymic carcinomas metastasize hematogeneously.

Reference

Freundlich IM, McGavaran MH: Abnormalities of the thymus. *J Thorac Imaging* 11:58-65, 1996.

Cross-Reference

Thoracic Radiology: THE REQUISITES, pp 432-435.

Comment

The differential diagnosis of this poorly marginated, soft tissue attenuation, anterior mediastinal mass includes a thymic neoplasm, lymphoma, and germ cell neoplasm. Lymphoma is typically associated with lymph node enlargement elsewhere, and germ cell neoplasms such as a mature teratoma frequently have evidence of fat attenuation or calcium.

Thymic neoplasms, most notably thymoma, account for the majority of anterior mediastinal masses in adult patients. Most thymic neoplasms demonstrate well-defined margins on imaging studies. Two notable exceptions are invasive thymoma and thymic carcinoma. Invasive thymoma refers to a thymoma that has invaded its fibrous capsule. Such lesions tend to spread locally, with invasion of adjacent mediastinal structures, chest wall invasion, and contiguous spread along the pleural surface (usually unilaterally). Thymic carcinoma is a rare thymic neoplasm that may be indistinguishable from an invasive thymoma on imaging studies unless distant metastases are present. Unlike invasive thymoma, a thymic carcinoma tends to metastasize hematogenously.

Notes

Subcarinal Lymph Node Enlargement Secondary to Metastatic Disease

1. Subcarinal lymph node enlargement, bronchogenic cyst, and left atrial enlargement.

2. Subcarinal lymph node enlargement.

3. Genitourinary, head and neck, breast, and skin (melanoma).

4. Azygoesophageal interface.

Reference

Libshitz HI: Intrathoracic lymph nodes. In: Freundlich IM, Bragg DG, Eds: *A Radiologic Approach to Diseases of the Chest*. Baltimore, Williams & Wilkins, 1992, pp 100-114.

Cross-Reference

Thoracic Radiology: THE REQUISITES, pp 440-441, 467-478.

Comment

The chest radiograph reveals a subcarinal mass, with associated lateral convex bulging of the azygoesophageal interface. The differential diagnosis of a subcarinal mass includes subcarinal lymph node enlargement, bronchogenic cyst, and left atrial enlargement. The MRI reveals that the mass is not vascular and has intermediate signal intensity similar to skeletal muscle. The MR features are thus most suggestive of lymph node enlargement. In this patient, the enlarged nodes were secondary to metastatic disease from a primary renal cell carcinoma.

Enlarged mediastinal lymph nodes may be encountered in a wide variety of neoplastic, infectious, and inflammatory conditions. Neoplastic causes include metastatic disease (from bronchogenic carcinoma or an extrathoracic primary), lymphoma, and leukemia. Infectious causes include tuberculosis (TB), fungal, viral, and bacterial infections. Although lymph node enlargement may be evident on CT images in the latter two entities, it is not usually evident on conventional radiographs. Inflammatory causes include sarcoidosis, Castleman's disease, and angioimmunoblastic lymphadenopathy.

Notes

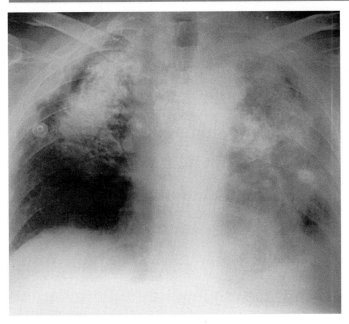
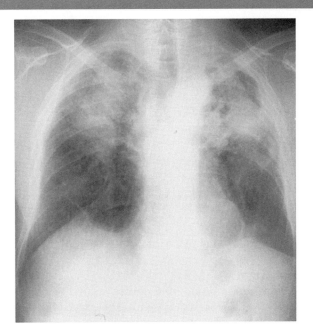

1. What term is used to describe the confluent areas of lung opacification observed in these two patients?

2. What pneumoconiosis is associated with this finding?

3. Is this finding typical of the simple or complicated form of this pneumoconiosis?

4. What term is used to describe the calcification pattern of the lymph nodes in the first figure?

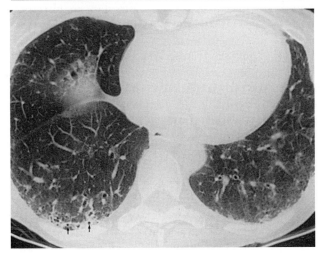
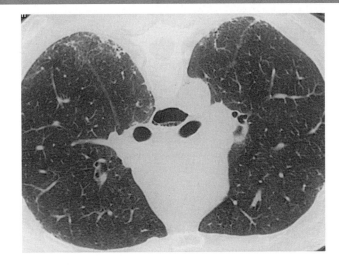

1. What is the distribution of lung abnormalities on these high-resolution CT (HRCT) images?

2. Name at least three causes of chronic infiltrative lung disease that are associated with a basilar and subpleural distribution of abnormalities.

3. Considering the presence of esophageal dilation, what is the most likely cause for this pattern of chronic infiltrative lung disease?

4. What soft tissue abnormality might you expect to see in a patient with this diagnosis?

C A S E 3 6

Silicosis

1. Progressive massive fibrosis.

2. Silicosis.

3. Complicated.

4. Eggshell calcification.

Reference

Stark P, Jacobsen F, Shaffer K: Standard imaging in silicosis and coal worker's pneumoconiosis. *Radiol Clin North Am* 30:1147-1154, 1992.

Cross-Reference

Thoracic Radiology: THE REQUISITES, pp 228-232.

Comment

Silicosis is a fibrotic lung disease related to the inhalation of dust containing either free crystalline silica or silicon dioxide. Occupational settings related to silica exposure include heavy metal mining, sandblasting, foundry work, and stone masonry. Silicosis is usually a slowly progressive chronic lung disease with a latency period of at least 20 years.

Chronic silicosis is classified into simple and complicated forms. Simple silicosis is asymptomatic and typically presents radiographically with multiple small, nodular opacities, ranging in size from 1 to 10 mm in diameter. The nodules usually have an upper lung zone predominance and frequently calcify. Enlarged nodes are often present and may demonstrate a characteristic peripheral eggshell pattern of calcification, as shown in the first figure.

Complicated silicosisis is associated with symptoms and reduced pulmonary function. It is characterized by one or more areas in which silicotic nodules have become confluent, measuring more than 1 cm in size. Such opacities may be observed in the periphery of the upper lung zone or in the middle lung zone. Over time, these opacities migrate toward the hila, with residual emphysema in the remaining portions of the lungs. In both figures, note the large vertically oriented opacities in the upper and middle lung zones, which are typical of the complicated form of silicosis. As progressive massive fibrosis becomes more extensive, the nodularity in the remaining portions of the lungs usually becomes less apparent.

Notes

C A S E 3 7

Interstitial Fibrosis Secondary to Scleroderma

1. Subpleural and basilar.

2. Idiopathic pulmonary fibrosis, interstitial lung disease associated with collagen vascular disorders, drug toxicity, and asbestosis.

3. Scleroderma.

4. Calcinosis.

Reference

Müller NM, Colby TV: Idiopathic interstitial pneumonias: high-resolution CT and histologic findings. *Radiographics* 17:1016-1022, 1997.

Cross-Reference

Thoracic Radiology: THE REQUISITES, pp 256-257.

Comment

The HRCT images demonstrate a subpleural distribution of irregular linear opacities, ground-glass attenuation, and traction bronchiolectasis. The last term refers to the small, discrete, cystic lucencies in the lung periphery (best demonstrated in the right lower lobe in the first figure [*arrows*]), which represent dilated bronchioles. A subpleural and basilar predominance of infiltrative lung disease is characteristic of usual interstitial pneumonia (UIP).

UIP is characterized histologically by a variegated pattern composed of foci of normal lung, interstitial cellular infiltrates, and intervening zones of active fibrosis and end-stage fibrosis. UIP is associated with a variety of chronic infiltrative lung diseases, including idiopathic pulmonary fibrosis, asbestosis, connective tissue disorders, and drug toxicity. Characteristic HRCT findings in patients with UIP include irregular linear opacities, ground-glass attenuation, traction bronchiectasis and bronchiolectasis, and honeycombing. Such findings typically demonstrate a subpleural and basilar predominance.

Scleroderma, also referred to as progressive systemic sclerosis, is a connective tissue disorder that is characterized by fibrosis and atrophy of numerous organ systems, including the skin, lungs, gastrointestinal tract, heart, and kidneys. Pulmonary manifestations include interstitial fibrosis, pulmonary vascular disease, and pleural thickening. Other common manifestations include esophageal dilation and dysmotility, enlarged mediastinal lymph nodes, and calcinosis in the skin and subcutaneous tissues. Although the interstitial lung abnormalities in this case are indistinguishable from those of other causes of UIP, the identification of esophageal dilation makes scleroderma the most likely diagnosis.

Notes

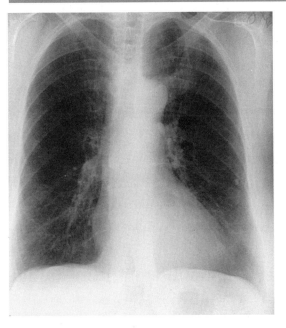 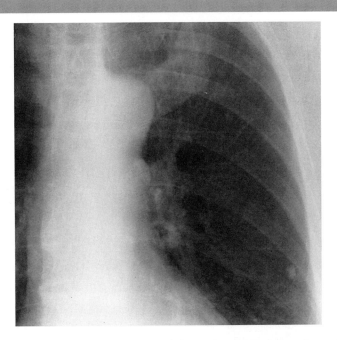

1. What term is used to describe the combination of a calcified lung nodule and calcified lymph nodes?
2. Are these findings more closely associated with primary or reactivation TB?
3. What does the term *Ghon focus* refer to?
4. Name the two most common radiographic findings associated with primary TB infection.

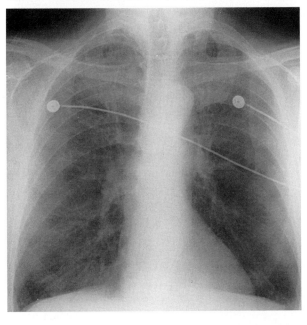 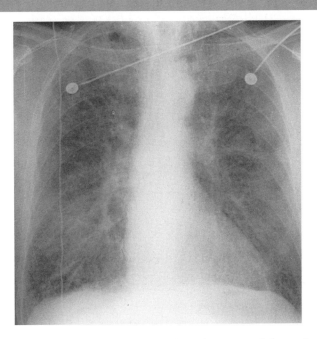

1. What is the most likely cause for the acute interstitial process demonstrated in the second figure?
2. What is the différence between Kerley A lines and Kerley B lines?
3. At approximately what pulmonary venous wedge pressure (PVWP) would you expect to detect Kerley lines?
4. Name at least three radiographic signs of interstitial edema.

C A S E   3 8

Ranke Complex

1. Ranke complex.

2. Primary.

3. A lung nodule that occurs at the initial site of parenchymal involvement from primary TB.

4. Parenchymal consolidation and mediastinal and hilar lymph node enlargement.

Reference

Leung AN: Pulmonary tuberculosis: the essentials. *Radiology* 210:307–322, 1999.

Cross-Reference

Thoracic Radiology: THE REQUISITES, pp 113–121.

Comment

Parenchymal consolidation and mediastinal and hilar lymph node enlargement are the hallmark of primary TB. The term *Ghon lesion* (or *Ghon focus*) refers to a lung nodule that is a residuum of primary TB. In patients with primary TB and an adequate host immune response, the area of lung consolidation slowly regresses to form a well-circumscribed nodule. Such a nodule may disappear altogether or may remain as a solitary calcified granuloma, referred to as a Ghon lesion. Lymph node enlargement, another sign of primary TB infection, also regresses. Residual calcified lymph nodes may be seen, as demonstrated in the aorticopulmonary window and left hilum in this patient.

Notes

C A S E   3 9

Interstitial Edema

1. Interstitial edema.

2. Kerley A lines are centrally located, radiate from the hila, and measure 2 to 6 cm in length; Kerley B lines are peripherally located, usually extend to the pleural surface, and measure less than 2 cm in length.

3. Higher than 17 mm Hg.

4. Peribronchial cuffing, indistinct pulmonary vessels; septal thickening (Kerley lines), and thickening of the fissures.

Reference

Hansell DM, Peters AM: Pulmonary vascular diseases and pulmonary edema. In: Armstrong P, Wilson AG, Dee P, Hansell DM, Eds: *Imaging of Diseases of the Chest*, second edition. St. Louis, Mosby, 1995, pp 369–425.

Cross-Reference

Thoracic Radiology: THE REQUISITES, pp 407–412.

Comment

The chest radiograph in the second figure demonstrates several typical findings of interstitial edema, including indistinctness of the pulmonary vessels, peribronchial cuffing, and thickened septal lines. The presence of a recent normal baseline radiograph confirms that this is an acute process. Significant ancillary findings include interval slight increase in heart size and increased caliber of upper lobe vessels (cephalization).

Cardiogenic pulmonary edema refers to excess extravascular fluid within the lungs secondary to increased pulmonary microvascular pressure, which is usually due to diseases of the left side of the heart such as left ventricular failure. Cardiogenic pulmonary edema usually follows a typical course. It begins in the interstitial compartment and extends into the alveolar compartment as it increases in severity.

The characteristic radiographic findings of pulmonary venous hypertension and congestive heart failure have been shown to correlate with physiologic parameters such as the PVWP. Normally, the PVWP is lower than 12 mm Hg. As PVWP rises to between 13 and 17 mm Hg, you should expect to see vascular redistribution. At PVWP higher than 17 mm Hg, Kerley lines are usually visible. At PVWP values higher than 20 mm Hg, a right-sided pleural effusion is often evident. When PVWP rises above 25 mm Hg, you should expect to see airspace opacities, usually most prominent in the central, perihilar regions of the lungs.

The chest radiographic features may lag behind the clinical status of the patient as pulmonary edema resolves. Radiographic findings of pulmonary edema may persist despite a return to normal wedge pressure measurements.

Notes

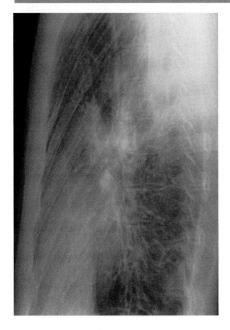

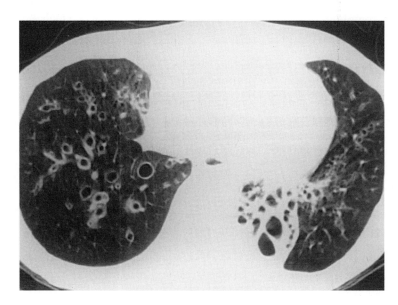

1. What airway abnormality is present in this patient?
2. What is the most common cause of this abnormality?
3. What conventional radiographic sign of bronchiectasis is evident in the lung bases in the first figure?
4. Name at least three CT findings associated with bronchiectasis.

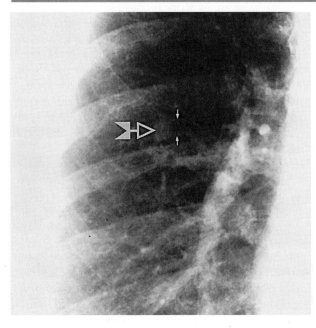

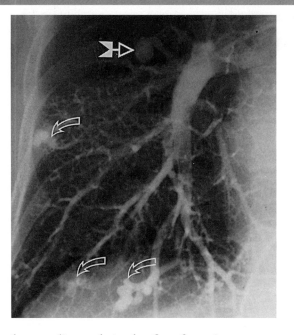

1. What is the etiology of the nodule shown on the chest radiograph in the first figure?
2. What syndrome is associated with pulmonary arteriovenous malformations (AVMs)?
3. Roughly what percentage of AVMs are multiple?
4. Name at least three symptoms or conditions that may be associated with a pulmonary AVM.

Bronchiectasis in a Patient With Marfan's Syndrome

1. Bronchiectasis.

2. Prior infection.

3. "Tram-tracking" (bronchial wall thickening).

4. Bronchial diameter greater than adjacent arterial diameter, identification of bronchi in the lung periphery, lack of normal bronchial tapering, bronchial wall thickening, and strings or clusters of cysts ± air-fluid levels.

Reference

Kim JS, Müller NL, Park C, et al: Cylindrical bronchiectasis: diagnostic findings on thin-section CT. *AJR Am J Roentgenol* 168:751–754, 1997.

Cross-Reference

Thoracic Radiology: THE REQUISITES, pp 386–396.

Comment

Bronchiectasis is defined as abnormal, irreversible dilation of the bronchi. Bronchiectasis may arise secondary to a wide variety of congenital and acquired abnormalities. Cystic fibrosis is the most common associated congenital abnormality, and prior infection, especially childhood viral illnesses, is the most common acquired abnormality. Bronchiectasis is a rare complication of Marfan's syndrome. Note the characteristic elongated thorax of this patient on the lateral radiograph.

Chest radiographs are frequently normal in patients with mild degrees of bronchiectasis but may occasionally reveal parallel thickened bronchial walls, also referred to as a tram-track appearance. With cystic bronchiectasis, radiographs may reveal clusters of air-filled cysts, often with fluid levels. HRCT is highly sensitive and specific for diagnosing bronchiectasis. Findings include a bronchial wall diameter greater than its adjacent artery, identification of bronchi within the peripheral third of the lung, lack of normal bronchial tapering, bronchial wall thickening, and strings or clusters of cysts. Complications of bronchiectasis include recurrent infections, hemoptysis, mucoid impaction, and atelectasis (note the left lower lobe atelectasis in the second figure).

Notes

Multiple Arteriovenous Malformations (Hereditary Hemorrhagic Telangiectasia)

1. AVM.

2. Hereditary hemorrhagic telangiectasia (HHT), also known as *Osler-Weber-Rendu disease*, which is characterized by telangiectasias, AVMs and aneurysms in multiple organ systems (including pulmonary, gastrointestinal, cutaneous, and central nervous system).

3. Approximately 30%.

4. Cyanosis, dyspnea, stroke, and brain abscess.

Reference

Remy J, Remy-Jardin M, Giraud F, Wattinne L: Angioarchitecture of pulmonary arteriovenous malformations: clinical utility of three-dimensional helical CT. *Radiology* 191:657–664, 1994.

Cross-Reference

Thoracic Radiology: THE REQUISITES, pp 84–86.

Comment

The coned-down chest radiograph in the first figure shows a well-circumscribed lung nodule *(open arrow)* lateral to the right hilum. The pulmonary arteriogram in the second figure shows that the nodule *(open straight arrow)* opacifies with contrast. It also demonstrates a feeding artery and a draining vein. The findings are consistent with an AVM. Note the presence of several additional AVMs in the right lung *(open curved arrows)*.

An AVM represents an abnormal communication between the pulmonary arteries and veins in which there is absence of the capillary network that normally separates these vascular structures. This process results in a right-to-left shunt. Although many patients are asymptomatic at the time of initial presentation, complications of right-to-left shunting include cyanosis, dyspnea, stroke, and brain abscess.

Pulmonary AVMs have a lower lobe predominance, and they often occur in the medial third of the lung. AVMs are defined as simple when there is a single feeding artery and a single feeding vein; they are complex when there are two or more feeding arteries and two or more draining veins.

On chest radiographs, pulmonary AVMs appear as well-defined nodules, which often have lobulated contours. A feeding artery and draining vein can often be identified *(small arrows* in the first figure).

Pulmonary arteriography has traditionally been the modality of choice for defining the number, size, and angioarchiecture of these lesions. Recently, spiral CT with three-dimensional (3D) reformation has been shown to be equivalent to pulmonary arteriography for diagnosis.

Notes

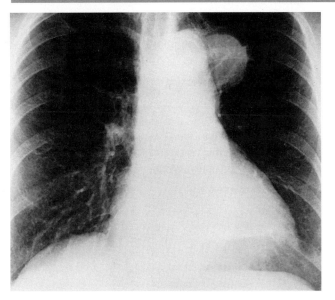
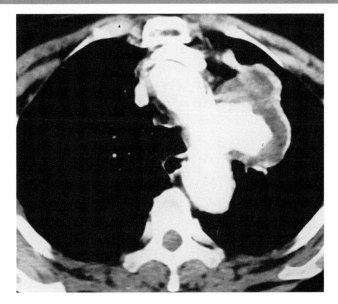

1. In which mediastinal compartment is this mass located?
2. What is the most likely diagnosis for this mass?
3. How would you characterize this aneurysm according to its shape?
4. Is this a typical location for an aneurysm associated with cystic medial necrosis?

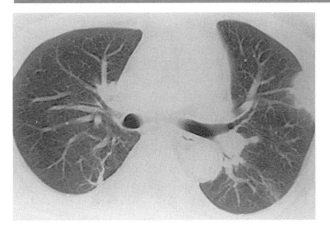
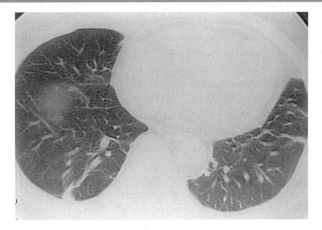

1. What is the differential diagnosis for the wedge-shaped, peripheral consolidation in the left lung in the first figure?
2. What is the significance of the identification of a feeding vessel directed toward the apex of the consolidation?
3. What is the significance of the linear bands that are present in both lower lobes?
4. What is the estimated prevalence of "incidentally detected" acute pulmonary embolism on contrast-enhanced spiral CT?

CASE 42

Saccular Aortic Aneurysm

1. Middle.

2. Aortic aneurysm.

3. Saccular.

4. No.

Reference

Naidich DP, Webb WR, Müller NL, et al: Aorta, arch vessels, and great veins. In: *Computed Tomography and Magnetic Resonance of the Thorax*, third edition. Philadelphia, Lippincott-Raven, 1999, pp 537–549.

Cross-Reference

Thoracic Radiology: THE REQUISITES, pp 447–449.

Comment

Vascular abnormalities, including aneurysms and vascular variants, are an important cause of middle mediastinal masses. You should consider the diagnosis of an aortic aneurysm whenever you detect a mass in close proximity to the aorta, particularly if a border of the mass is indistinguishable from the aortic contour. The diagnosis can be confirmed with either contrast-enhanced CT or MRI.

A thoracic aortic aneurysm is an abnormal dilation of the aorta, usually defined as greater than 4 cm in diameter. Aortic aneurysms can be classified according to shape, integrity of the aortic wall, and location. With regard to shape, aneurysms may be classified as either saccular or fusiform. Saccular aneurysms are characterized by a focal outpouching of the aorta, as demonstrated in the second figure. Such aneurysms are often infectious in etiology. Fusiform aneurysms, on the other hand, are characterized by cylindrical dilation of the entire aortic circumference. This configuration is typical of atherosclerotic aneurysms.

Based on the integrity of the aortic wall, aneurysms may be classified as either true or false. True aneurysms have an intact aortic wall. The most common cause of a true aneurysm is an atherosclerotic aneurysm. In contrast, false aneurysms are associated with a disrupted aortic wall. Examples of false aneurysms include infectious (mycotic) and posttraumatic aneurysms. Regarding location, aneurysms may be classified as involving primarily the ascending aorta, aortic arch, or descending aorta. Aneurysms that classically involve the ascending aorta include those related to cystic medial necrosis and syphilis. Other causes of aneurysms, including atherosclerotic, mycotic, and posttraumatic etiologies, most often affect the descending thoracic aorta and aortic arch.

Notes

CASE 43

Pulmonary Infarction

1. Pulmonary infarct, neoplasm, pneumonia, and hemorrhage.

2. A feeding vessel is a feature that is more typical of pulmonary infarction than the other entities listed in Answer 1.

3. Linear bands have been described as an ancillary lung parenchymal finding in patients with acute pulmonary embolism (PE).

4. Approximately 1% to 5%.

Reference

Coche, EE, Müller NL, Kim K, Wiggs BR, Mayo JR. Acute pulmonary embolism: ancillary findings at spiral CT. *Radiology* 207:753–758, 1998

Cross-Reference

Thoracic Radiology: THE REQUISITES, p 416.

Comment

Pulmonary infarcts typically appear as wedge-shaped foci of consolidation, with their bases abutting the visceral pleura. Like pulmonary emboli, they are usually multiple, and they typically have a basilar predominance.

Coche and associates recently reported two CT lung parenchymal findings that were significantly associated with acute PE: (1) wedge-shaped peripheral foci of consolidation and (2) linear bands. Although not specific for the diagnosis of PE, the identification of these findings, especially the former, should prompt a careful review of the pulmonary vasculature for vascular signs of acute PE. If CT is inconclusive for PE, these lung findings may suggest the need for additional diagnostic studies to exclude the diagnosis of PE.

Notes

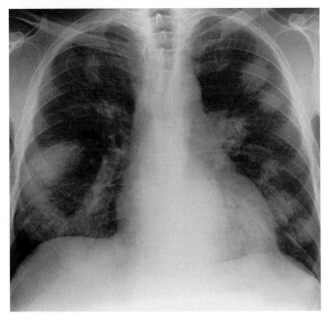
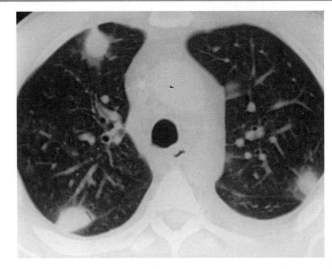

1. What is the differential diagnosis of multiple lung nodules or masses in a patient with acquired immunodeficiency syndrome (AIDS)?

2. In AIDS patients, is the doubling time of nodules a reliable way to differentiate between benign and malignant conditions?

3. What is the most common type of lymphoma to affect patients with AIDS?

4. Which nuclear medicine study can be used to distinguish Kaposi's sarcoma from lymphoma?

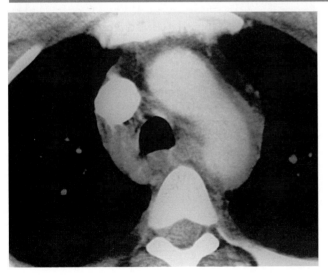
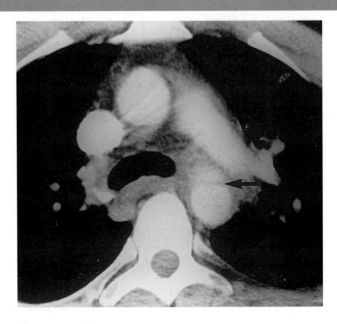

1. Name the three most common sites of traumatic aortic transection.

2. Of those patients who survive to reach the hospital, what is the most common site of injury?

3. Is a mediastinal hematoma specific for aortic injury?

4. What is the significance of periaortic mediastinal hemorrhage?

Acquired Immunodeficiency Syndrome–Related Lymphoma

1. Infection (fungal, mycobacterial, septic emboli) and neoplasm (lymphoma and Kaposi's sarcoma).

2. No.

3. Non-Hodgkin's lymphoma.

4. Gallium scan.

Reference

Lee VW, Fuller JD, O'Brien MJ, et al: Pulmonary Kaposi's sarcoma in patients with AIDS: scintigraphic diagnosis with sequential thallium and gallium scans. *Radiology* 180:409–412, 1991.

Cross-Reference

Thoracic Radiology: THE REQUISITES, pp 142–149.

Comment

Lymphoma is the second most common AIDS-related neoplasm (Kaposi's sarcoma is the most common), but thoracic involvement is present in only a minority of AIDS patients with non-Hodgkin's lymphoma. Thoracic lymphoma is usually associated with disseminated disease involving the central nervous system, gastrointestinal tract, and bone marrow. In AIDS patients, thoracic lymphoma is typically extranodal. Thus, abnormalities of the lung parenchyma (nodules, masses, interstitial parenchymal opacities) and pleura (effusions) are encountered more frequently than lymph node enlargement.

The differential diagnosis of multiple nodules or masses includes infections and other neoplasms, especially Kaposi's sarcoma. In AIDS-related lymphoma, nodules and masses may grow quite rapidly, with doubling times similar to that of infectious nodules. Thus, a rapid doubling time is not a reliable indicator of benignancy in AIDS patients. With regard to Kaposi's sarcoma, it can be differentiated from lymphoma by its lack of uptake on gallium scans. In contrast, lymphoma is gallium-avid.

Notes

Traumatic Aortic Transection

1. At the level of the ligamentum arteriosum, the aortic root, and the diaphragm.

2. The level of the ligamentum arteriosum.

3. No.

4. It is more specific for aortic injury.

Reference

Kuhlman JE, Pozniak MA, Collins J, Knisely BL: Radiographic and CT findings of blunt chest trauma: aortic injuries and looking beyond them. *Radiographics* 18:1085–1106, 1998.

Cross-Reference

Thoracic Radiology: THE REQUISITES, pp 193–196, 479–482.

Comment

Acute thoracic aortic injury is a serious complication of blunt chest trauma, with an associated high mortality rate. The majority of affected patients die before reaching the hospital, and approximately half of those who present to the hospital die within 24 hours.

Spiral CT is playing an increasingly important role in screening trauma patients for evidence of mediastinal hematoma, an important indirect sign of aortic injury. Although mediastinal hemorrhage is sensitive for detecting aortic injury, it is not very specific. For example, mediastinal hematoma may be associated with injuries to other arterial and venous structures, as well as with nonvascular injuries, such as sternal and spinal fractures. When hemorrhage is localized to the periaortic region (first figure), it is more specific for aortic injury.

Direct signs of aortic injury include deformity of the aortic contour (second figure), intimal flap (*arrow* in the second figure), intraluminal clot or debris, pseudoaneurysm, and frank extravasation of contrast. The role of CT in the diagnosis of aortic injury is evolving. Although a confident CT diagnosis of aortic injury (based on the presence of direct signs of aortic injury) is considered sufficient preoperative evaluation at some medical centers, angiographic confirmation is still required preoperatively at many other centers.

Notes

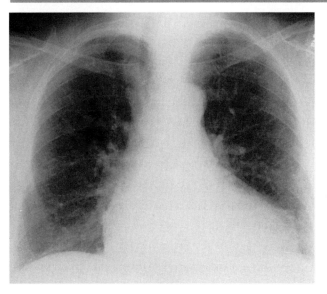
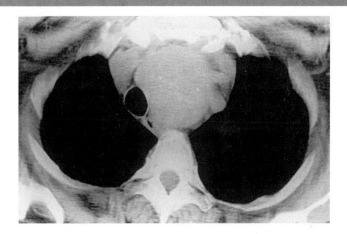

1. What is the most common cause of a thoracic inlet mediastinal mass in an adult patient?

2. What is the most common cause of a thoracic inlet mass in a child?

3. Which CT imaging feature of this mass makes untreated lymphoma a highly unlikely diagnosis?

4. Do thyroid goiters typically enhance with intravenous contrast?

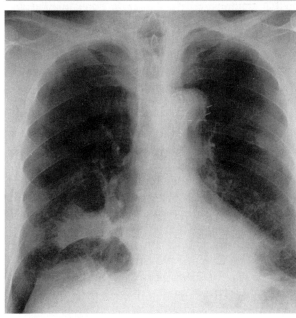
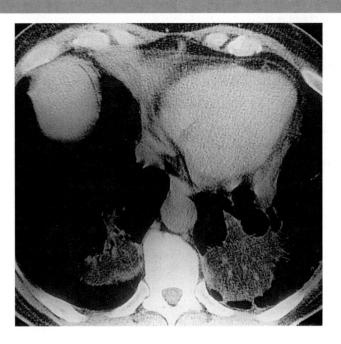

1. What is the most likely diagnosis?

2. Name four other causes of chronic airspace consolidation.

3. How can you differentiate this entity from the remaining causes of chronic consolidation?

4. What aspirated substance is most closely associated with this entity?

CASE 46

Thyroid Goiter

1. Thyroid goiter.

2. Lymphangioma.

3. The presence of calcification.

4. Yes.

Reference

Reed JC: Anterior mediastinal mass. In: *Chest Radiology: Plain Film Patterns and Differential Diagnoses,* fourth edition. St. Louis, Mosby–Year Book, 1997, pp 107–124.

Cross-Reference

Thoracic Radiology: THE REQUISITES, pp 432–439.

Comment

A thyroid goiter is the most common cause of a mediastinal mass in the thoracic inlet region in adults. On chest radiographs, a substernal goiter typically presents as a well-defined mass that extends through the thoracic inlet from the neck, and it is frequently associated with deviation and/or compression of the trachea. On CT imaging, characteristic features include continuity with the cervical thyroid gland, foci of high attenuation on noncontrast images (reflecting the high iodide content of thyroid tissue), focal areas of cysts and calcification, and intense enhancement following intravenous contrast administration.

Although lymphoma may infrequently present as a thoracic inlet mass, calcification is rarely encountered in untreated cases of lymphoma. In contrast, calcification is a common feature of thyroid goiters.

Notes

CASE 47

Lipoid Pneumonia

1. Lipoid pneumonia.

2. Bronchoalveolar cell carcinoma, alveolar proteinosis, lymphoma, and "alveolar" sarcoid (not a true alveolar process).

3. Only lipoid pneumonia is characterized by fat density on CT.

4. Mineral oil.

Reference

Kukafka DS, Kaplan MA, Criner GJ: A 77-year-old man with a lung mass. *Chest* 111:1439–1441, 1997.

Cross-Reference

Thoracic Radiology: THE REQUISITES, pp 280–281.

Comment

Exogenous lipoid pneumonia is associated with the inadvertent aspiration of oily substances such as mineral oil. On conventional radiographs, lipoid pneumonia typically appears as chronic alveolar consolidation, which is usually most prominent in the lung bases. Lipoid pneumonia infrequently presents as a focal mass-like opacity.

On CT examination, the areas of consolidation are characterized by low density, reflecting their fatty composition. The identification of negative CT density numbers in the range of fatty tissue (e.g., -50 to -150 Hounsfield units) within the consolidation is pathognomonic for lipoid pneumonia.

Affected patients are frequently asymptomatic, but a minority of patients present with chronic symptoms of cough and dyspnea. Such symptoms generally resolve once the patient discontinues using the offending substance.

With regard to the differential diagnosis of chronic alveolar consolidation, you may narrow the differential diagnosis by assessing whether the process is focal or diffuse. Focal areas of chronic consolidation may be seen in lipoid pneumonia, bronchoalveolar cell carcinoma (BAC), and lymphoma. Diffuse chronic consolidation can be seen in BAC, alveolar proteinosis, alveolar sarcoid, and lipoid pneumonia. Lipoid pneumonia typically has a dependent distribution, which is not typical of other causes of chronic diffuse alveolar consolidation.

Notes

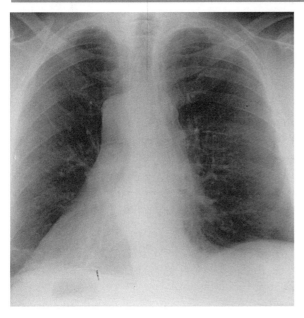 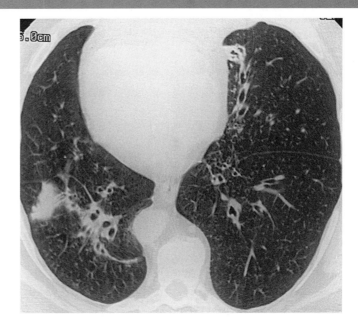

1. What is the most likely diagnosis?
2. What is the classic triad of abnormalities associated with this entity?
3. Name one other manifestation that affects male patients with this disorder.
4. What is the pattern of inheritance?

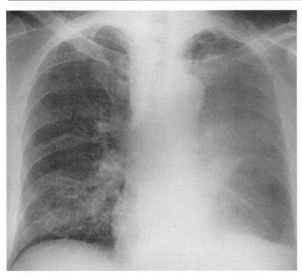 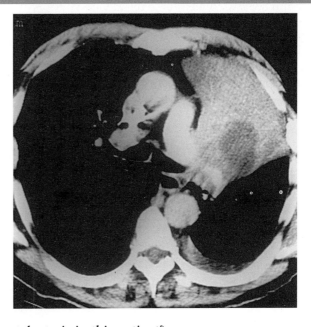

1. What is the most likely cause of left upper lobe atelectasis in this patient?
2. How can you differentiate the obstructing mass from the adjacent atelectatic lung in this case?
3. Based solely on the degree of postobstructive atelectasis present, what is the correct T stage for this non-small cell lung cancer?
4. If the pleural effusion is proven malignant, what would be the correct T stage for this patient?

C A S E 4 8

Kartagener's Syndrome

1. Kartegener's syndrome.

2. Situs invertus, bronchiectasis, and sinusitis.

3. Infertility.

4. Autosomal recessive.

Reference

Wilson AG: Diseases of the airways. In: Armstrong P, Wilson AG, Dee P, Hansell DM, Eds: *Imaging of Diseases of the Chest*, second edition. St. Louis, Mosby, 1995, p 835.

Cross-Reference

Thoracic Radiology: THE REQUISITES, pp 394–395.

Comment

Kartagener's syndrome is a subset of the dyskinetic cilia syndrome, a congenital cause of bronchiectasis that is associated with an autosomal recessive pattern of inheritance. In patients with the dyskinetic cilia syndrome, ciliary function is typically abnormal throughout the body. Thus, affected males are infertile on the basis of immotile sperm.

Patients with Kartagener's syndrome typically present in childhood with symptoms related to bronchitis, sinusitis, and rhinitis. Bronchiectasis usually develops in childhood and young adulthood, and it is associated with recurrent pneumonias. Bronchiectasis is typically less severe than in cases of cystic fibrosis, another congenital cause of bronchiectasis. Interestingly, in patients with Kartagener's syndrome, bronchiectasis has a predilection for the anatomic right middle lobe.

On imaging studies, the combination of situs inversus and bronchiectasis suggests the diagnosis. Ancillary findings may include overinflation of the lungs and focal areas of consolidation and atelectasis.

Notes

C A S E 4 9

Left Upper Lobe Collapse Secondary to Bronchogenic Carcinoma

1. Bronchogenic carcinoma.

2. The necrotic tumor mass enhances to a lesser degree than the atelectatic lung.

3. T2.

4. T4.

Reference

Jett J, Feins R, Kvale P, et al: Pretreatment evaluation of non-small cell lung cancer. *Am J Respir Crit Care Med* 156:320–332, 1997.

Cross-Reference

Thoracic Radiology: THE REQUISITES, pp 37–41, 316–323.

Comment

The most common cause of complete lobar atelectasis is obstruction of a central bronchus. In an adult patient, bronchogenic carcinoma is the most likely diagnosis.

The TNM classification system is used for staging non-small cell lung cancer. According to this classification system, a centrally obstructing neoplasm with associated postobstructive atelectasis or pneumonia involving less than an entire lung is classified as T2. If the entire lung is involved, then the primary tumor is classified as T3.

A malignant pleural effusion is classified as T4, a status that is considered inoperable disease. Although a pleural effusion in the setting of lung cancer is often indicative of pleural metastases, in some cases an effusion may be sympathetic or parapneumonic. Therefore, if the status of the pleural effusion will alter patient management, cytopathologic proof of malignancy is mandatory.

Notes

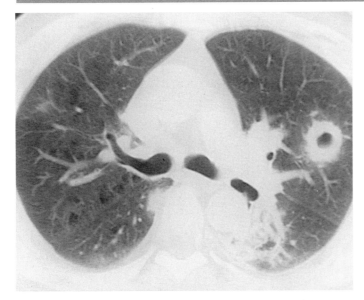

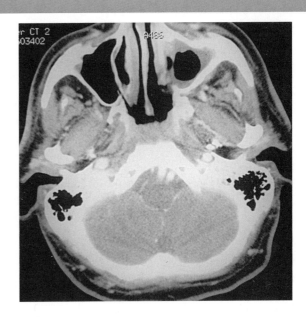

1. What is the most likely diagnosis?

2. What other organ system is frequently involved by this disorder?

3. Does this patient have the "limited" form of this disorder?

4. What laboratory test is most helpful for confirming this diagnosis?

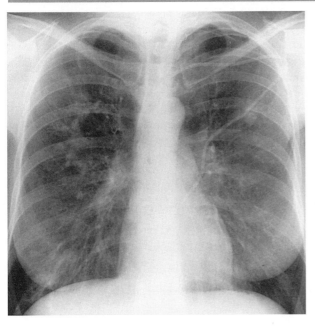

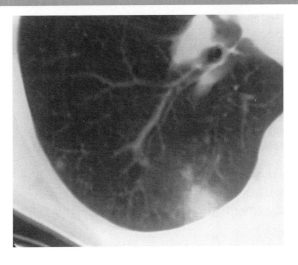

1. Which form of *Aspergillus* infection typically presents with multiple poorly defined lung nodules?

2. Is the "CT-halo sign" (a "halo" of ground-glass opacification surrounding a nodule) specific for *Aspergillus*?

3. What does the ground glass surrounding the nodule represent?

4. Is the CT-halo sign typically seen early or late in the course of infection with *Aspergillus*?

Wegener's Granulomatosis

1. Wegener's granulomatosis.

2. Renal.

3. No.

4. Cytoplasmic pattern of antineutrophil cytoplasmic autoantibody (cANCA).

Reference

Frazier AA, Rosado-de-Christenson ML, Galvin JR, Fleming MV: Pulmonary angiitis and granulomatosis: radiologic-pathologic correlation. *Radiographics* 18:687–710, 1998.

Cross-Reference

Thoracic Radiology: THE REQUISITES, p 262.

Comment

Wegener's granulomatosis is a necrotizing vasculitis that classically involves the upper respiratory tract, lungs, and renal glomeruli. A limited form of the disease is largely confined to the lung and is associated with a better prognosis than the classic form.

The thoracic radiologic manifestations of Wegener's granulomatosis are varied, but the most characteristic pattern is that of multiple lung nodules or masses. Such nodules and masses are usually round in configuration, with well-defined margins. They range from 1 or 2 mm to 9 cm in diameter, and cavitation is evident in up to one half of cases. On CT scans, the nodules frequently demonstrate angiocentric features, such as the presence of feeding vessels and a peripheral distribution. The second most common pattern is focal or diffuse alveolar consolidation, which corresponds to the presence of pulmonary hemorrhage.

The diagnosis requires consistent pathologic, radiologic, clinical, and laboratory data. The presence of a cytoplasmic pattern of cANCA, as detected by indirect immunofluorescence of serum, is suggestive of the diagnosis. Treatment with a combination of cyclophosphamide and steroids is successful in most cases.

Notes

Invasive *Aspergillus*

1. Invasive.

2. No.

3. Hemorrhage.

4. Early.

Reference

Connolly JE, McAdams HP, Erasmus JJ, Rosado-de-Christenson ML: Opportunistic fungal pneumonia. *J Thorac Imaging* 14:51–62, 1999.

Cross-Reference

Thoracic Radiology: THE REQUISITES, p 137.

Comment

Invasive pulmonary aspergillosis is the most common fungal infection to affect immunosuppressed patients. It usually affects patients with severe neutropenia, including recent bone marrow transplant recipients, patients with hematologic malignancies, and patients receiving high-dose steroids. Because it is a potentially lethal infection, prompt recognition and treatment are critical.

Aspergillus organisms invade blood vessels, resulting in areas of pulmonary infarction. On chest radiographs, you may observe multiple poorly defined nodular opacities and more confluent areas of consolidation. When imaged with CT scanning early in the course of infection, the nodules typically demonstrate a halo of ground-glass attenuation, which corresponds to the presence of hemorrhage. In the proper clinical setting (e.g., profound neutropenia), the CT halo sign is highly suggestive of *Aspergillus* infection. However, it is not specific for *Aspergillus*, because it may also be seen in association with other infections (mucormycosis), vasculitides, and hemorrhagic metastases. Later in the course of infection, the nodules may undergo cavitation (the "air crescent sign"). Such cavitation occurs after granulocyte recovery and usually indicates a good prognosis.

Notes

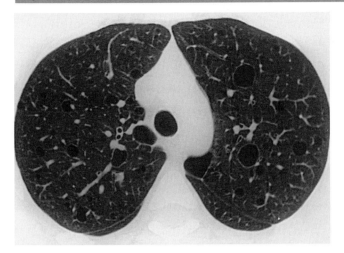 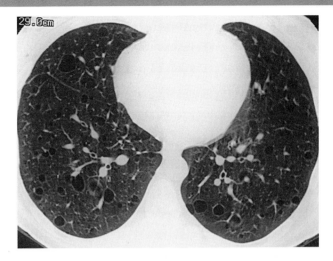

1. Name two infiltrative lung diseases that are associated with a cystic pattern.

2. Describe the typical demographic features (age, sex) of a patient with lymphangioleiomyomatosis (LAM).

3. Is LAM associated with cigarette smoking?

4. Name two pleural complications of LAM.

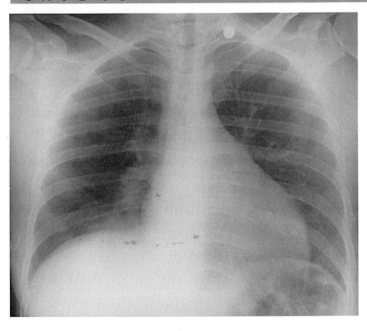 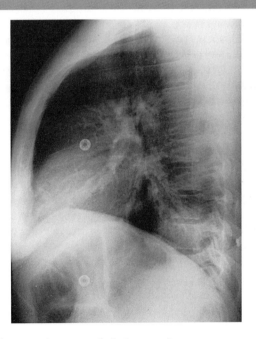

1. What is the most likely cause of focal consolidation in a human immunodeficiency virus (HIV)–positive patient?

2. What is the second most common cause?

3. How often does *Pneumocystis carinii* pneumonia (PCP) present with this pattern?

4. Are recurrent bacterial pneumonias an AIDS-defining illness?

Lymphangioleiomyomatosis

1. LAM and eosinophilic granuloma.

2. Young (reproductive age) female.

3. No.

4. Pneumothorax and chylothorax.

Reference

Sullivan EJ: Lymphangioleiomyomatosis: a review. *Chest* 114:1689-1703, 1998.

Cross-Reference

Thoracic Radiology: THE REQUISITES, pp 220-222.

Comment

LAM is a rare disease that exclusively affects women, predominately during their reproductive years. Pathologically, it is characterized by abnormal proliferation of immature smooth muscle cells. Obstruction of bronchioles results in the development of thin-walled lung cysts. Such cysts may rupture, leading to spontaneous pneumothoraces. Lymphatic obstruction may result in chylous pleural effusions.

On conventional radiographs, you may observe a diffuse linear pattern, with preserved or increased lung volumes. Pleural abnormalities, including pneumothorax and pleural effusion, may also be evident. The hallmark of LAM on HRCT is the presence of numerous thin-walled cysts, which are usually regular and uniform in configuration. The intervening lung is typically normal.

The main differential diagnosis is histiocytosis X. In this disorder, cysts are usually accompanied by small nodules, which may undergo cavitation. Unlike the cysts in LAM, histiocytosis X–related cysts have a more variable appearance, with occasional bizarre configurations. Finally, histiocytosis X typically spares the costophrenic sulci, whereas LAM has a more diffuse distribution.

Notes

Community-Acquired Bacterial Pneumonia

1. Community-acquired bacterial pneumonia.

2. Tuberculosis.

3. In approximately 10% of cases.

4. Yes.

Reference

Boiselle PM, Tocino I, Hooley RJ, et al: Chest radiograph interpretation of *Pneumocystis carinii* pneumonia, bacterial pneumonia, and pulmonary tuberculosis in HIV-positive patients: accuracy, distinguishing features, and mimics. *J Thorac Imaging* 12:47-53, 1997.

Cross-Reference

Thoracic Radiology: THE REQUISITES, pp 142-145.

Comment

The chest radiograph plays an important role in the evaluation of pulmonary infections in HIV-positive patients. Despite some overlapping features among various infections, chest radiograph pattern recognition can help effectively narrow the differential diagnosis of pulmonary infections in HIV-positive patients.

With regard to a pattern of focal or lobar consolidation, bacterial pneumonia is the most likely etiology. Bacterial pneumonias are especially common early in the course of HIV infection (CD4 >200/mm³), and recurrent bacterial pneumonias are now included as an AIDS-defining illness. Commonly encountered bacterial pathogens include *Streptococcus*, *Haemophilus influenzae*, *Staphylococcus*, and gram-negative organisms.

When focal or lobar consolidation is accompanied by mediastinal and hilar lymph node enlargement, TB should be considered. Other causes of focal or lobar consolidation are less common, including PCP (which more typically presents as diffuse, bilateral parenchymal opacities) and *Mycobacterium avium-intracellulare* infection.

Notes

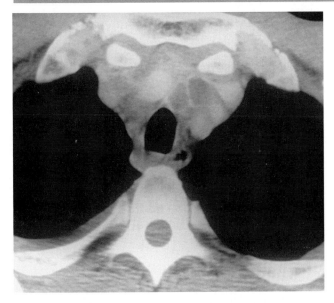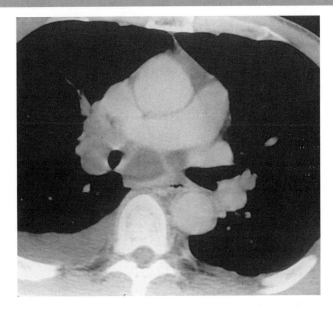

1. What infection is most closely associated with low-density nodes with peripheral enhancement?

2. Is lymph node enlargement more common in primary TB or reactivation TB?

3. In patients with primary TB, is lymph node enlargement more common in pediatric or adult patients?

4. Concerning HIV-positive patients and TB, are enlarged mediastinal lymph nodes encountered more commonly in patients with CD4 counts above 200/mm³ or in patients with CD4 counts below 200/mm³?

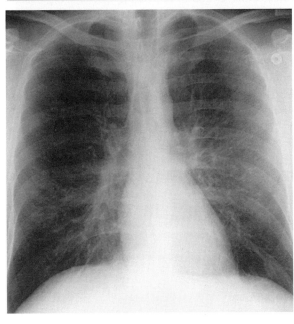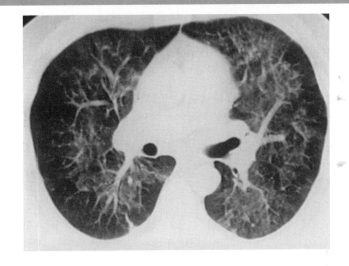

1. In an HIV-positive patient, what is the most likely diagnosis for these findings?

2. Is PCP increasing or decreasing in prevalence among HIV-positive patients in the United States?

3. Below what CD4 count level are patients at risk for PCP?

4. Does a normal chest radiograph exclude PCP?

Tuberculosis

1. Tuberculosis.

2. Primary TB.

3. Pediatric.

4. CD4 counts below 200/mm³.

Reference

Leung AN: Pulmonary tuberculosis: the essentials. *Radiology* 210:307–322, 1999.

Cross-Reference

Thoracic Radiology: THE REQUISITES, pp 113–121, 441.

Comment

Lymph node enlargement is a characteristic feature of primary TB, particularly in children. Lymph node enlargement may occur alone or in association with parenchymal consolidation. On contrast-enhanced CT scans of patients with mediastinal tuberculous lymphadenitis, enlarged nodes often demonstrate a low-density center and peripheral rim enhancement. Histologically, such nodes have been shown to demonstrate central necrosis and a highly vascular, inflammatory capsular reaction.

Although low-density nodes are characteristic of TB, they are not specific for this entity. Such nodes may also be encountered in atypical mycobacterial and fungal infections. Neoplastic lymph nodes (e.g., metastatic seminoma) may also demonstrate this appearance.

With regard to TB in HIV-positive patients, the radiographic appearance varies depending on the patient's CD4 count. In patients with CD4 counts above 200/mm³, a reactivation pattern is typically seen. In patients with CD4 counts below 200/mm³, you will usually observe a primary pattern, including low-density lymph nodes and consolidation.

Notes

Pneumocystis carinii Pneumonia

1. PCP.

2. Decreasing (secondary to improved prophylaxis).

3. CD4 <200/mm³.

4. No.

Reference

McGuinness G: Changing trends in the pulmonary manifestations of AIDS. *Radiol Clin North Am* 35:1029–1082, 1997.

Cross-Reference

Thoracic Radiology: THE REQUISITES, pp 142–145.

Comment

The classic chest radiographic presentation of PCP is a bilateral perihilar or diffuse symmetric interstitial pattern, which may be finely granular, reticular, or ground glass in appearance. Importantly, the chest radiograph may be normal at the time of presentation in a significant minority of cases of PCP. CT, particularly HRCT, is more sensitive than chest radiographs for detecting PCP and thus may be helpful in evaluating symptomatic patients with normal or equivocal radiographic findings.

The classic CT finding in PCP is extensive ground-glass attenuation, which corresponds to the presence of intraalveolar exudate, consisting of fluid, organisms, and debris. It is often distributed in a patchy or geographic fashion, with a predilection for the central, perihilar regions of the lungs. Ground-glass attenuation is occasionally accompanied by thickened septal lines, and foci of consolidation may also be evident in severe cases. In up to a third of cases of PCP, ground-glass opacities are accompanied by cystic lung disease. Such cysts have an upper lobe predominance and demonstrate varying sizes and wall thicknesses.

Notes

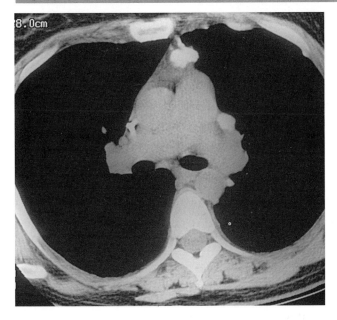 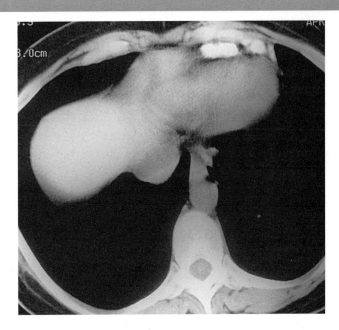

1. Name four benign causes of calcified lymph nodes.

2. In patients with lymphoma, are calcified lymph nodes usually seen before or after radiation therapy?

3. Name a neoplasm that can result in ossified lymph nodes.

4. Which lymph node group is involved in the second figure?

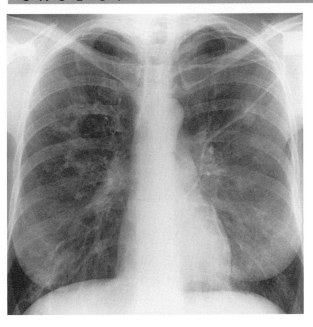 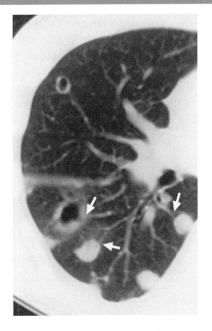

1. Name two types of infections that may result in rapidly growing nodules in a non-AIDS immunosuppressed patient.

2. What organism is most closely associated with septic infarcts?

3. Name two common sources of septic infarcts.

4. List four CT features of septic infarcts.

C A S E 5 6

Ossified Lymph Nodes Secondary to Metastatic Osteosarcoma

1. Tuberculosis, histoplasmosis, sarcoidosis, and silicosis.

2. After.

3. Osteosarcoma.

4. Superior diaphagmatic nodes.

Reference

Johnson GL, Askin FB, Fishman EK: Thoracic involvement from osteosarcoma: typical and atypical CT manifestations. *AJR Am J Roentgenol* 168:347–349, 1997.

Cross-Reference

Thoracic Radiology: THE REQUISITES, p 441.

Comment

Calcified lymph nodes are usually benign, and they are often related to granulomatous processes, such as TB, histoplasmosis, or sarcoidosis. Neoplastic causes of calcified lymph nodes are less common. They include metastases from mucinous adenocarcinomas and lymphoma. With regard to lymphoma, calcification is frequently seen following radiation therapy, but it is rarely encountered in untreated cases.

Ossified lymph nodes are a rare manifestation of metastatic osteosarcoma. Such nodes appear similar to calcified lymph nodes. In patients with osteosarcoma, the presence of lymph node metastases portends a poor prognosis. Lymphatic involvement is usually accompanied by metastases within the lung, a common site of metastases. Lung metastases frequently demonstrate ossification.

Notes

C A S E 5 7

Septic Infarcts

1. Fungal *(Aspergillus, Mucor)*; septic infarcts.

2. *Staphylococcus aureus*.

3. Tricuspid endocarditis (often seen in intravenous drug abusers) and indwelling catheters and prosthetic devices.

4. Poorly defined nodules that frequently cavitate, wedge-shaped foci of consolidation, peripheral and basilar predominance, and feeding vessel.

Reference

Kuhlman JE, Fishman EK, Teigen C. Pulmonary septic emboli: diagnosis with CT. *Radiology* 174:211–213, 1990.

Cross-Reference

Thoracic Radiology: THE REQUISITES, p 96.

Comment

Septic infarcts most often originate from right-sided tricuspid endocarditis or from infected thrombi within systemic veins. On chest radiographs and CT scans of patients with septic infarcts, you may observe poorly defined nodular opacities and areas of wedge-shaped parenchymal opacification. Such opacities are usually peripheral in location, and they have a predilection for the lower lobes. Cavitation is frequently observed, particularly on CT scans. A characteristic finding on CT scans is the identification of feeding vessels leading to the nodules (*arrows* in the second figure) and wedge-shaped parenchymal opacities. Thus, the CT finding of cavitating nodules with feeding vessels is highly suggestive of septic infarcts.

Notes

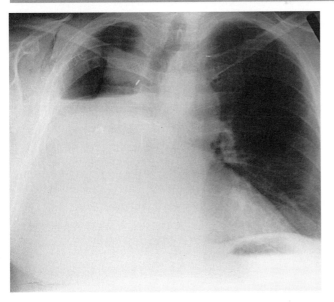
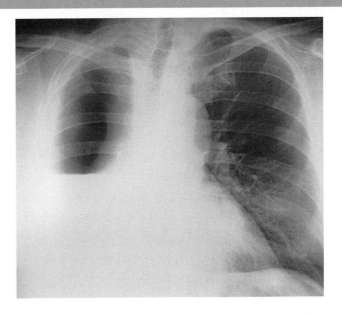

1. What postoperative complication is evident in this case (the first radiograph was obtained prior to the second)?

2. Is bronchopleural fistula more common following left- or right-sided pneumonectomy?

3. List four radiographic signs of bronchopleural fistula following pneumonectomy.

4. What nuclear medicine study can be helpful in confirming this diagnosis?

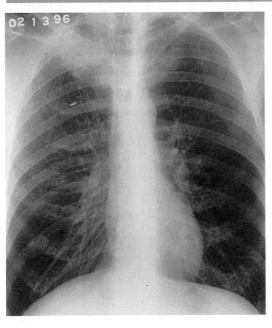
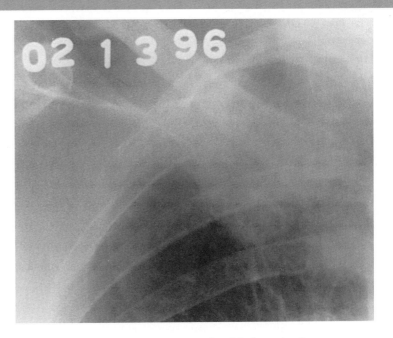

1. What is the most common cell type of bronchogenic carcinoma to present in this location?

2. Does the presence of chest wall invasion make this an inoperable lesion?

3. Neoplastic involvement of which three structures would preclude resection of this mass?

4. What imaging modality is best suited for determining the resectability of a superior sulcus tumor?

Bronchopleural Fistula

1. Bronchopleural fistula.

2. Right-sided.

3. Failure of the pneumonectomy space to fill with fluid; abrupt decrease in the air-fluid level in the pneumonectomy space; contralateral shift of the mediastinum following pneumonectomy; and identification of air in a previously completely opacified pneumonectomy space.

4. Xenon ventilation study.

Reference
Tsukada G, Stark P: Postpneumonectomy complications. *AJR Am J Roentgenol* 169:1363–1370, 1997.

Cross-Reference
None.

Comment
Bronchopleural fistula is a relatively uncommon but serious complication following pneumonectomy, with a prevalence of 5% and a mortality rate of roughly 20%. Major predisposing factors relate to operative causes of bronchial ischemia, such as a long bronchial stump, too proximal a ligation of the bronchial arteries, and disruption of bronchial blood supply from extensive lymph node dissection. Additional risk factors include preoperative radiation therapy, steroid therapy, malnutrition, and resection through tumor or infection.

Following pneumonectomy, the mediastinum is normally shifted toward the side of resection, and the pneumonectomy space gradually fills with fluid over time. Bronchopleural fistula should be considered when any of the following are observed: (1) the pneumonectomy space fails to fill with fluid; (2) there is an abrupt decrease in the air-fluid level in the pneumonectomy space; (3) there is a new collection of air in a previously opacified pneumonectomy space; or (4) there is contralateral shift of the mediastinum. The diagnosis can be confirmed with a xenon ventilation study, which will demonstrate xenon activity in the pneumonectomy space.

Notes

Superior Sulcus Tumor

1. Squamous cell carcinoma.

2. No.

3. Vertebral body, subclavian artery, or brachial plexus.

4. MRI.

Reference
Arcasoy SM, Jett JR: Superior pulmonary sulcus tumors and Pancoast's syndrome. *N Engl J Med* 19:1370–1376, 1997.

Cross-Reference
Thoracic Radiology: THE REQUISITES, p 319.

Comment
A bronchogenic carcinoma arising at the extreme apex of the lung is referred to as a superior sulcus tumor. Affected patients typically present with symptoms of shoulder pain, Horner's syndrome (ptosis, miosis, anhidrosis), and weakness and atrophy of intrinsic muscles of the hand.

MRI is more accurate than CT for determining the resectability of a superior sulcus tumor. Superior sulcus neoplasms may be considered resectable if there is no involvement of the vertebral body, brachial plexus, or subclavian artery. Note the presence of rib destruction adjacent to the mass (best visualized on the coned-down image), indicative of chest wall invasion. Chest wall invasion does not preclude surgical resection of a superior sulcus tumor.

Operable candidates are usually treated with preoperative radiation followed by surgery with chest wall resection. The overall 5-year survival for such patients is between 20% and 35%.

Notes

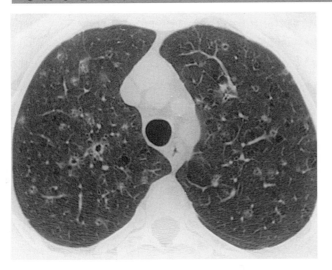
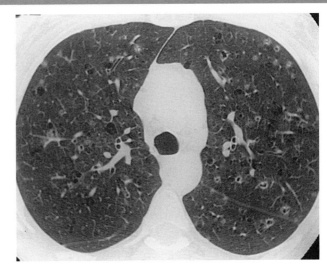

1. What is the most likely cause for these HRCT findings?
2. Approximately what percentage of patients with this disorder are cigarette smokers?
3. In patients with histiocytosis X, which portion of the lungs is usually spared?
4. Would you expect this patient to have diminished lung volumes?

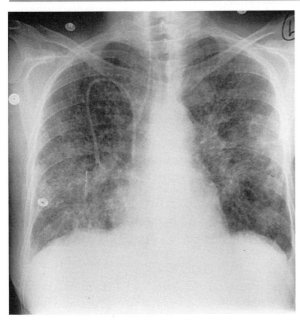
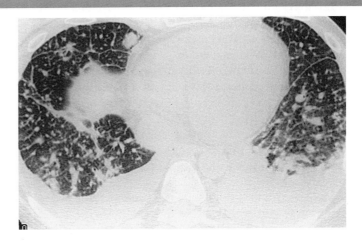

1. Name three possible diagnoses for the chest radiograph findings in this patient with breast cancer who is receiving chemotherapy.
2. Based on the HRCT findings, which diagnosis is most likely?
3. Name four primary neoplasms that are commonly associated with lymphangitic carcinomatosis.
4. Which primary neoplasm is most closely associated with a unilateral distribution of lymphangitic carcinomatosis?

CASE 60

Histiocytosis X

1. Histiocytosis X.

2. Approximately 90%.

3. Costophrenic angles.

4. No.

Reference

Brauner M, Grenier P, Tijani K, Battesti JP, Valeyre D: Pulmonary Langerhans cell histiocytosis: evolution of lesions on CT scans. *Radiology* 204:497–502, 1997.

Cross-Reference

Thoracic Radiology: THE REQUISITES, p 222.

Comment

Histiocytosis X is an uncommon idiopathic disorder that is characterized histologically by the benign proliferation of mature histiocytes. In its early stages, histiocytosis X is characterized by the presence of multiple granulomatous nodules, which are often peribronchiolar in distribution. In later stages of the disease, the nodules are replaced by cysts.

Affected patients are usually young and middle-aged adults, and there is a strong association with cigarette smoking. Symptoms include dyspnea and dry cough.

On conventional radiographs, you may observe a reticulonodular pattern, with the upper lobes affected to a greater degree than the lower lobes. The costophrenic angles are typically spared. Lung volumes are usually normal or increased.

On HRCT, you may observe small nodules, which are typically centrilobular and peribronchiolar in distribution. Such nodules may undergo cavitation, and they may eventually form thin-walled cysts. Cysts associated with histiocytosis X are less uniform in appearance than cysts associated with LAM. Because nodules are not a feature of LAM, the identification of both nodules and cysts should suggest the diagnosis of histiocytosis X.

Notes

CASE 61

Lymphangitic Spread of Neoplasm

1. Lymphangitic carcinomatosis, atypical infection, and drug toxicity.

2. Lymphangitic carcinomatosis.

3. Colon, lung, breast, and stomach.

4. Lung.

Reference

Munk PL, Müller NL, Miller RR, Ostrow DN: Pulmonary lymphangitic carcinomatosis: CT and pathologic findings. *Radiology* 166:705–709, 1988.

Cross-Reference

Thoracic Radiology: THE REQUISITES, pp 216–218.

Comment

Pulmonary lymphangitic carcinomatosis refers to tumor growth within the lymphatics of the lungs. Interestingly, most lymphangitic metastases are thought to arise from hematogenous spread. Lymphangitic carcinomatosis occurs most commonly in patients with carcinoma of the colon, lung, breast, stomach, and adenocarcinoma of unknown primary.

The chest radiographic findings of lymphangitic carcinomatosis are nonspecific. They include diffuse reticulonodular or linear opacities, septal lines, hilar and mediastinal lymph node enlargement, and pleural effusions.

The HRCT findings of lymphangitic carcinomatosis are more specific. The observed abnormalities reflect the distribution of lymphatics within the lung: (1) smooth or nodular axial interstitial thickening along the bronchovascular bundles; (2) smooth or nodular septal thickening; (3) smooth or nodular thickening of the fissures; and (4) identification of polygonal structures (secondary pulmonary lobules). An important ancillary observation is the preservation of normal lung architecture. The differential diagnosis for these HRCT findings includes lymphoma, sarcoidosis, and Kaposi's sarcoma.

Notes

CASE 62

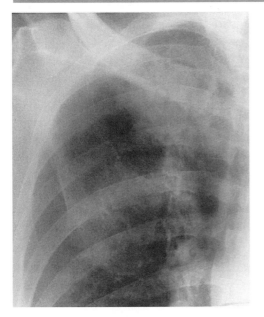
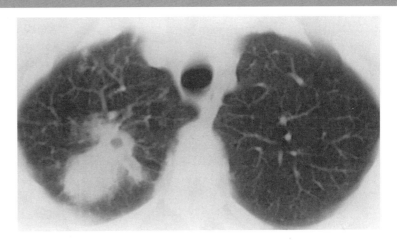

1. What is the most likely diagnosis for these imaging findings?
2. What are "satellite" nodules?
3. What is their significance?
4. What are the most common sites for reactivation TB in the lung?

CASE 63

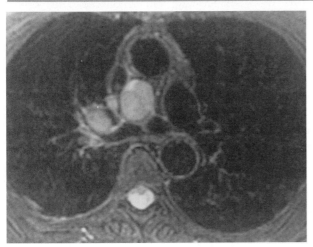
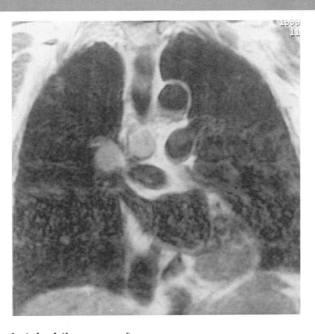

1. What is the most likely cause of the precarinal and right hilar masses?
2. Do MRI signal characteristics of lymph nodes effectively distinguish between benign and malignant lymph nodes?
3. Is MRI more accurate than CT in the assessment of mediastinal lymph nodes in patients with lung cancer?
4. Is MRI more accurate than CT in the detection of hilar lymph nodes?

Reactivation Tuberculosis

1. Tuberculosis.

2. Small, often rounded, opacities that lie in close proximity to a larger nodule or mass.

3. They are more suggestive of an infectious process, such as TB, rather than a lung carcinoma.

4. Apical and posterior segments of the upper lobes and superior segments of the lower lobes.

Reference

Leung AN: Pulmonary tuberculosis: the essentials. *Radiology* 210:307–322, 1999.

Cross-Reference

Thoracic Radiology: THE REQUISITES, pp 114–119.

Comment

The chest radiograph demonstrates a poorly marginated mass in the right lung apex, without evidence of calcification. CT is often helpful to further characterize a lung nodule or mass. In this case, CT reveals a focus of cavitation that is not apparent on the conventional radiograph. There are also two important ancillary findings on the CT image. First, there are several small nodules adjacent to the mass. Such nodules are referred to as satellite nodules, and their presence suggests an infectious etiology, such as TB, rather than a lung carcinoma. Second, note the presence of numerous small, centrilobular, linear and branching, Y- and V-shaped opacities, a pattern that is also referred to as tree-in-bud. This pattern is often associated with bronchogenic spread of TB, a type of dissemination that occurs when a cavity erodes into an adjacent airway. Thus, the combination of an apical lung cavity, satellite nodules, and a tree-in-bud pattern is highly suggestive of reactivation TB.

Notes

Mediastinal and Hilar Lymph Node Enlargement in a Patient With Bronchogenic Carcinoma

1. Mediastinal and hilar lymph node enlargement.

2. No.

3. No.

4. Yes.

Reference

Boiselle PM, Patz EF, Vining DJ, Weissleder R, Shepard JO, McLoud TC: Imaging of mediastinal lymph nodes: CT, MR, and FDG PET. *Radiographics* 18:1061–1069, 1998.

Cross-Reference

Thoracic Radiology: THE REQUISITES, pp 440–442.

Comment

Lymph node enlargement is a common cause of a mediastinal or hilar mass and should be suspected whenever a spherical or ovoid mass or masses is identified within a known anatomic lymph node location. There are a variety of infectious, inflammatory, and neoplastic causes of thoracic lymph node enlargement.

Neoplastic etiologies include bronchogenic carcinoma, metastatic disease, and lymphoma. This patient has a bronchogenic carcinoma in the right upper lobe (not shown on these images), and the lymph nodes were proven malignant at biopsy.

Both CT and MRI rely on anatomic features of lymph nodes, most notably lymph node size (short axis > 1 cm), to distinguish between malignant and benign lymph nodes. This strategy is limited by a low sensitivity and specificity. Thus, in patients with bronchogenic carcinoma, enlarged nodes must be biopsied for staging purposes.

MRI is more accurate than CT in the detection of hilar nodes. In most cases, however, CT provides a satisfactory assessment of both mediastinal and hilar lymph node enlargement. MRI is reserved as a secondary, problem-solving tool for inconclusive CT cases.

Notes

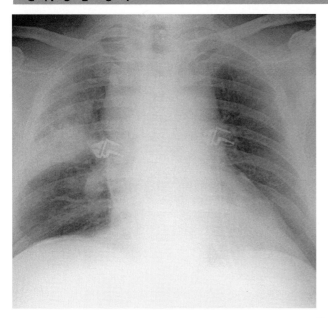 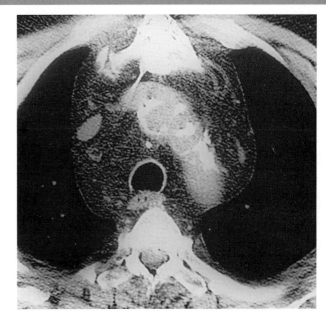

1. What is the cause of diffuse mediastinal widening in this patient?
2. Does this disorder require therapy?
3. Name three risk factors for developing this condition.
4. Where does excess fat usually accumulate in patients with this condition?

C A S E 6 4

Mediastinal Lipomatosis

1. Mediastinal lipomatosis.

2. No.

3. Cushing's syndrome, steroid therapy, and obesity.

4. Anterior and superior mediastinum, cardiophrenic angles, and paravertebral and retrocrural regions.

Reference

Naidich DP, Zerhouini EA, Seigelman SS, Eds: *Computed Tomography and Magnetic Resonance of the Thorax*. New York, Raven, 1991, pp 60–61.

Cross-Reference

Thoracic Radiology: THE REQUISITES, pp 463–465.

Comment

The chest radiograph demonstrates a right upper lobe pneumonia and diffuse mediastinal widening. There are a variety of causes of mediastinal widening, including mediastinal lipomatosis, mediastinitis, diffuse mediastinal lymphadenopathy, and mediastinal hemorrhage. The widened mediastinum is relatively symmetric in appearance, and there is no deviation of the trachea. Such features are typical of mediastinal lipomatosis, but a definitive diagnosis requires demonstration of fat by CT or MRI. The CT image confirms the diagnosis of mediastinal lipomatosis.

Mediastinal lipomatosis refers to the diffuse accumulation of excess unencapsulated fat within the mediastinum. Fat accumulation is usually most prominent in the anterior and superior portions of the mediastinum. Fat may also accumulate in other parts of the mediastinum, including the cardiophrenic angles and the paravertebral region. An important diagnostic feature is the homogeneous appearance of the mediastinal fat. A heterogeneous appearance should raise the suspicion of another superimposed process, such as mediastinal hemorrhage or neoplastic infiltration of the mediastinal fat.

Notes

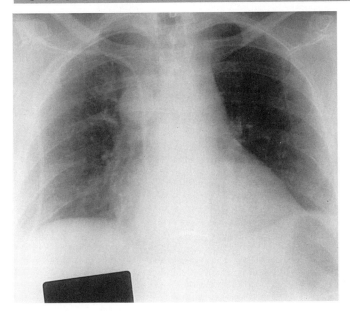
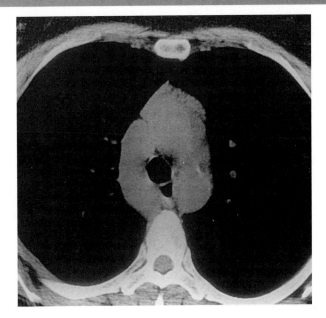

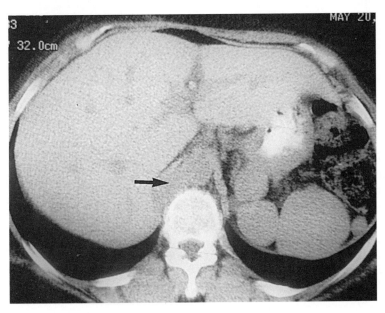

1. What congenital vascular abnormality is evident in this case?
2. Which mediastinal interface is typically displaced in patients with this condition?
3. Name an associated extravascular abnormality that is present on the CT image of the abdomen.
4. Name at least two additional causes of azygos vein enlargement.

Azygos Continuation of the Inferior Vena Cava

1. Azygos continuation of the inferior vena cava.

2. Azygoesophageal interface.

3. Polysplenia.

4. Obstruction of the vena cava, tricuspid insufficiency, and right-sided heart failure.

Reference
Naidich DP, Zerhouini EA, Seigelman SS, Eds: *Computed Tomography and Magnetic Resonance of the Thorax*. New York, Raven, 1991, pp 47–50.

Cross-Reference
Thoracic Radiology: THE REQUISITES, pp 455–456.

Comment
The chest radiograph and thoracic CT image demonstrate marked distention of the arch of the azygos vein. The abdominal CT image shows dilation of the retrocrural portion of the azygos vein *(arrow)* and absence of a definable inferior vena cava. The constellation of findings is diagnostic of azygos continuation of the inferior vena cava, a congenital anomaly that is associated with both the asplenia and polysplenia syndromes. Note multiple spleens in the left upper quadrant of the abdomen on the abdominal CT image.

On chest radiographs of affected patients, you will observe widening of the azygos arch contour and displacement of the azygoesophageal recess below this level. CT can confirm the diagnosis by demonstrating absence of a definable inferior vena cava. CT is also helpful in excluding other causes of azygos vein distention such as obstruction of the vena cava.

Notes

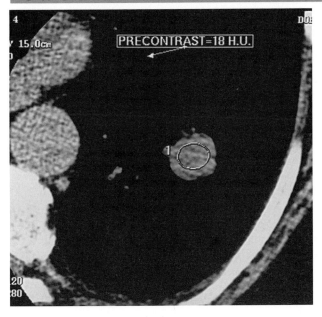
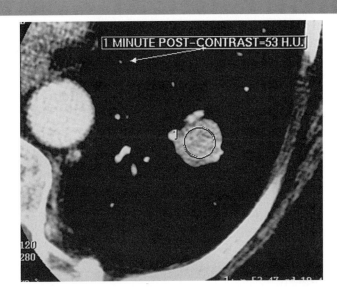

1. How would you describe the margins of this nodule?
2. Pre-contrast and 1-minute post-contrast images demonstrate nodule enhancement of 35 Hounsfield units. Is this degree of enhancement diagnostic of a benign entity?
3. Which noninvasive test has a higher specificity for malignancy: FDG-PET or CT pulmonary nodule enhancement?
4. Does CT pulmonary nodule enhancement have a high or low negative predictive value for malignancy?

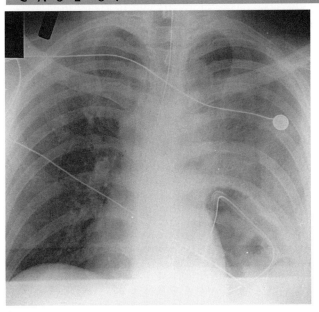
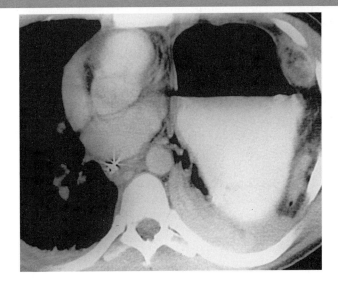

1. Which hemidiaphragm is more often affected by tramautic rupture, the left or the right?
2. What are the two most common causes of diaphragm rupture?
3. In patients with traumatic rupture of the left hemidiaphragm, which organ is most commonly herniated?
4. Name five radiographic signs of left hemidiaphragm rupture.

CT Pulmonary Nodule Enhancement

1. Lobulated.

2. No.

3. FDG-PET.

4. High negative predictive value.

Reference

Swensen SJ, Viggiano RW, Midthun DE, et al: Lung nodule enhancement at CT: multicenter study. *Radiology* 214:73–80, 2000.

Cross-Reference

Thoracic Radiology: THE REQUISITES, pp 340–343.

Comment

The CT images demonstrate a lung nodule with lobulated margins, which enhances by 35 Hounsfield units. The degree of enhancement is greater than the 15 Hounsfield unit threshold for this test and is thus of concern for a malignant process.

CT pulmonary nodule enhancement is a relatively new, noninvasive technique that relies on the principle that malignant nodules are generally more vascular than benign nodules, such as granulomas. This technique requires meticulous attention to the study protocol described by Swensen and colleagues. The protocol employs the use of serial spiral CT acquisitions (3 mm collimation) before and at four sequential 1-minute intervals following the intravenous administration of contrast. Nodule enhancement values are obtained by placing a region of interest measurement within the nodule center. Enhancement less than 15 Hounsfield units is highly predictive of a benign process (negative predictive value for malignancy is 96%). Enhancement greater than 15 Hounsfield units is of concern for malignancy, but the specificity is only moderate (58%). Such enhancing nodules generally require further assessment, such as biopsy or surgical resection.

It is important to be aware that there are specific nodule requirements for this protocol. Nodules should be relatively spherical in shape and homogeneous in appearance, without evidence of necrosis, calcification, cavitation, or fat. Moreover, patients should be able to perform reproducible breath-holds.

Notes

Traumatic Rupture of the Left Hemidiaphragm

1. Left.

2. Blunt trauma and penetrating injury.

3. Stomach.

4. Nasogastric tube coiled in the thorax, apparent elevation of the hemidiaphragm with loss of its normal dome shape, changing hemidiaphragm levels on serial radiographs, contralateral mediastinal shift, and left pleural effusion.

Reference

Shackleton KL, Stewart ET, Taylor AJ: Traumatic diaphragmatic injuries: spectrum of radiographic findings. *Radiographics* 18:49–59, 1998.

Cross-Reference

Thoracic Radiology: THE REQUISITES, pp 188–193.

Comment

Diaphragmatic rupture is an uncommon but serious complication of blunt and penetrating trauma. The left hemidiaphragm is affected more often than the right side. The left-sided predominance is thought to be secondary to two factors: a protective effect from the liver on the right side, and relative weakness of the left hemidiaphragm compared with the right.

Because of the morbidity and mortality from associated bowel obstruction and strangulation, a prompt diagnosis of diaphragm rupture is important. Unfortunately, however, the diagnosis is often delayed. You should suspect this diagnosis when you observe apparent elevation of a hemidiaphragm, changing hemidiaphragm levels on serial radiographs, or an unusual contour of the hemidiaphragm. A more specific finding is the identification of stomach or bowel in the thorax. CT or MRI can confirm the diagnosis. Because of its multiplanar imaging capability and superb visualization of the diaphragm, MRI is the preferred method of diagnosis. However, spiral CT is better suited for the evaluation of clinically unstable patients with suspected diaphragm rupture.

Notes

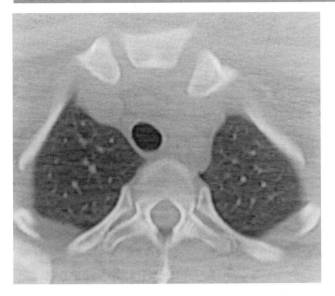
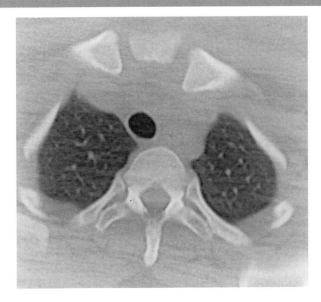

1. What skeletal injury is evident on these CT images?

2. Which is more common—anterior or posterior dislocation?

3. Name a potential complication of posterior dislocation.

4. What is the best method for establishing or confirming a diagnosis of sternoclavicular joint dislocation?

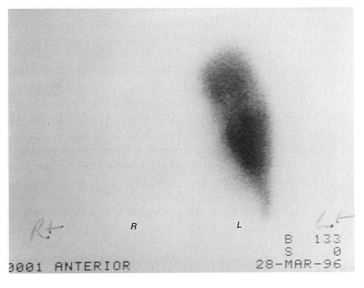
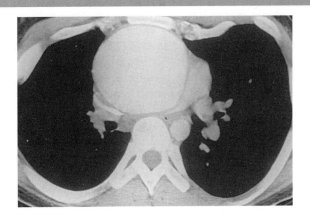

1. Is pulmonary embolus the most common cause of unilateral absent perfusion on a VQ scan?

2. What is the cause in this case?

3. What entities are associated with ascending aortic aneurysms?

4. What other aortic abnormality can result in this scintigraphic appearance?

Posterior Sternoclavicular Joint Dislocation

1. Left posterior sternoclavicular joint dislocation.

2. Posterior.

3. Injury to the brachiocephalic or subclavian veins.

4. CT.

Reference

Harris JH, Harris WH, Novelline RA, Eds: Chest. In: *The Radiology of Emergency Medicine.* Baltimore, Williams & Wilkins, 1993, pp 498-500.

Cross-Reference

None.

Comment

Sternoclavicular joint dislocation is a relatively uncommon injury that is usually associated with massive direct trauma to the anterior chest wall. Affected patients typically present with a large hematoma of the upper anterior chest wall and asymmetry of the clavicles on palpation.

The diagnosis can be difficult to make on portable chest radiographs, because only minimal displacement is usually evident on such studies. Moreover, the sternoclavicular joints are often altered in appearance radiographically on the basis of patient rotation. When this injury is suspected on the basis of clinical or radiographic findings, a limited CT study through the level of the sternoclavicular joints can readily establish the diagnosis. In the setting of a posterior dislocation, CT also provides an assessment of the brachiocephalic and subclavian veins for signs of injury.

Notes

Right Pulmonary Artery Compression by Ascending Aortic Aneurysm

1. No.

2. Ascending aortic aneurysm.

3. Connective tissue disorders (Marfan's and Ehlers-Danlos syndromes) and syphilis.

4. Aortic dissection.

Reference

Pickhardt PJ, Fischer KC: Unilateral hypoperfusion or absent perfusion on pulmonary scintigraphy: differential diagnosis. *AJR Am J Roentgenol* 171:145-150, 1998.

Cross-Reference

Thoracic Radiology: THE REQUISITES, pp 447-449.

Comment

A variety of entities may result in the presence of unilateral absence of perfusion on pulmonary scintigraphy scans. Interestingly, thromboembolism accounts for only a minority of such cases. Nonthromboembolic causes include mediastinal and hilar masses, ascending aortic aneurysm and dissection, pulmonary artery hypoplasia and agenesis, pulmonary artery sarcoma, and pneumonectomy. When confronted with this pattern on a pulmonary scintigraphy study, you should carefully assess the chest radiograph for the presence of a nonthromboembolic cause, such as a central mass. CT is often helpful for further evaluation, because it can readily distinguish between an intrinsic filling defect of the pulmonary artery and an extrinsic compression of the vessel.

In this case, absent perfusion to the right lung is caused by severe compression of the right pulmonary artery by an ascending aortic aneurysm. Ascending aortic aneurysms are usually associated with connective tissue disorders such as Marfan's and Ehlers-Danlos syndromes. Syphilis is an infrequent cause of ascending aortic aneurysm. Right pulmonary artery compression is an uncommon complication of ascending aortic aneurysm. More common complications include rupture, dissection, aortic insufficiency, and pericardial tamponade.

Notes

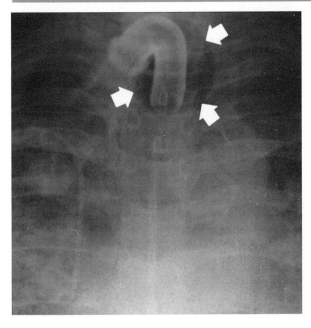

1. What does the circular lucency *(arrows)* adjacent to the tracheostomy tube represent?
2. Name at least two potential complications of an overinflated tracheostomy tube or endotracheal tube cuff.
3. Name two types of fistulas that may occur as a tracheostomy tube complication.
4. What is the ideal location for the tip of a tracheostomy tube?

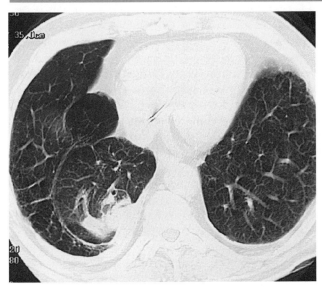 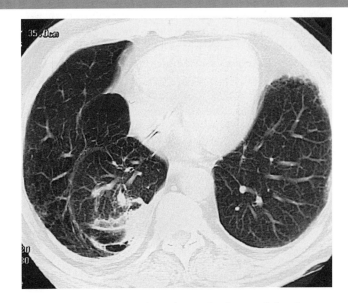

1. What is the most likely cause for the parenchymal abnormality observed in the right lower lobe in this patient?
2. Name the term that is used to describe the whorled appearance of the adjacent bronchovascular bundles.
3. What occupational exposure is most closely related to this process?
4. Is rounded atelectasis associated only with asbestos-related pleural disease?

CASE 70

Overinflated Tracheostomy Tube Cuff

1. An overinflated tracheostomy tube cuff.

2. Tracheal stricture, tracheomalacia, tracheal rupture, and tracheoesophageal fistula.

3. Tracheoesophageal and tracheoarterial.

4. The tip should ideally be positioned halfway between the stoma and the carina.

Reference

Stark P: Imaging of tracheobronchial injuries. *J Thorac Imaging* 10:206–219, 1995.

Cross-Reference

Thoracic Radiology: THE REQUISITES, pp 351–352.

Comment

A tracheostomy tube is usually placed for long-term ventilatory support or to establish an airway distal to the presence of a laryngeal obstruction. Most long-term complications of intubation relate to cuff injury. In recent years, the advent of low-pressure, high-volume cuffs has been associated with a decreased rate of cuff complications.

If the cuff is overinflated, blood supply to the mucosa of the trachea is compromised, leading to ischemic necrosis. Late complications of ischemic necrosis include tracheal stricture and tracheomalacia.

A second mechanism of airway injury relates to abnormal angulation of the tube. This problem occurs more frequently with tracheostomy tubes than with endotracheal tubes. Angulation of the tube can result in erosion, ulceration, and eventual perforation of the tracheal wall. Posterior angulation can lead to a tracheoesophageal fistula, and anterolateral angulation can result in a tracheoarterial fistula with either the innominate or the carotid artery. Rarely, an overinflated cuff can directly erode a vessel and result in a tracheoarterial fistula. In this particular case, an overinflated cuff resulted in a tracheocarotid fistula, which proved fatal.

Notes

CASE 71

Rounded Atelectasis

1. Rounded atelectasis.

2. The "comet tail sign."

3. Asbestos.

4. No.

Reference

Partap ZA: The comet tail sign. *Radiology* 213:553–554, 1999.

Cross-Reference

Thoracic Radiology: THE REQUISITES, pp 241–244.

Comment

Rounded atelectasis refers to a form of peripheral lobar collapse that develops in patients with pleural disease. Although it is most commonly associated with asbestos-related pleural disease, rounded atelectasis may occur in the setting of chronic pleural thickening from any etiology.

On chest radiography, it typically appears as a round or oval, sharply marginated mass that occurs most commonly in the lower lobes. The mass usually abuts an area of pleural thickening, which is usually greatest in dimension near the mass. The mass forms acute angles with the adjacent lung parenchyma and is usually separated from the diaphragm by interposed aerated lung.

A characteristic feature of rounded atelectasis is the presence of a curvilinear tail, which has been referred to as the comet tail sign. This refers to the presence of crowded bronchi and blood vessels that extend from the lower border of the mass to the hilum, creating a whorled appearance of the bronchovascular bundle. Signs of volume loss are occasionally evident on chest radiography but are usually minimal. On CT examinations, displacement of the adjacent fissure is frequently observed.

In this case, the CT findings of a focal parenchymal opacity adjacent to an area of pleural thickening with associated volume loss and a comet tail sign are diagnostic of rounded atelectasis. For cases in which the CT findings are equivocal, fine-needle aspiration biopsy is suggested to exclude malignancy because of the high association between bronchogenic carcinoma and asbestos exposure in smokers.

Notes

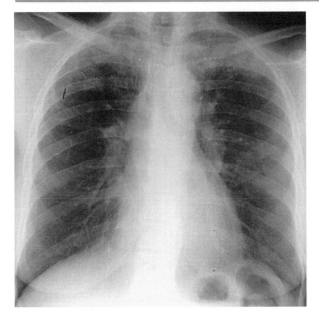

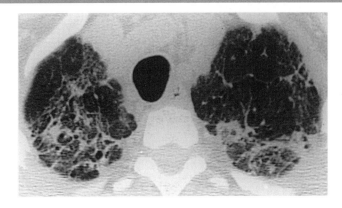

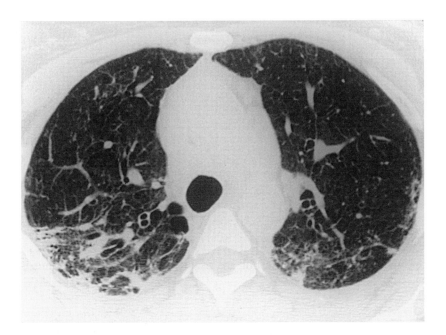

1. Name at least four causes of an upper zone distribution of chronic infiltrative lung disease.

2. Which of these entities is most closely associated with a reticular and nodular pattern on chest radiographs?

3. What is the term used to describe irregular bronchial dilation associated with pulmonary fibrosis?

4. What laboratory test is usually elevated in patients with sarcoidosis?

Sarcoidosis

1. Silicosis, coal worker's pneumoconiosis, sarcoidosis, ankylosing spondylitis, histiocytosis X, and chronic berylliosis.

2. Sarcoidosis.

3. Traction bronchiectasis.

4. Angiotensin-converting enzyme (ACE) levels.

Reference

Miller BH, Rosado-de-Christenson ML, McAdams HP, Fishback NF: Thoracic sarcoidosis: radiologic-pathologic correlation. *Radiographics* 15:421–437, 1995.

Cross-Reference

Thoracic Radiology: THE REQUISITES, pp 213–216.

Comment

The chest radiograph reveals a bilateral upper lung zone distribution of reticular and nodular opacities with associated upper lobe volume loss. The HRCT images in the second and third figures demonstrate irregular linear and small nodular opacities with associated architectural distortion and traction bronchiectasis and bronchiolectasis.

Among the various causes of an upper lung zone distribution of chronic infiltrative lung disease, sarcoidosis is most closely associated with a reticular and nodular pattern. Roughly 20% of sarcoid patients with evidence of interstitial lung disease will develop fibrosis. The fibrosis is usually most pronounced in the apical and posterior portions of the upper lobes (as demonstrated in this case) and in the superior segments of the lower lobes. Signs of volume loss and architectural distortion are commonly observed.

Notes

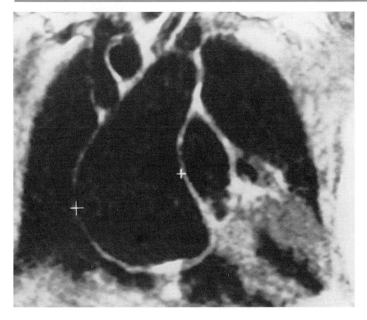

1. What vascular abnormality is evident on this MRI?
2. Name at least two entities that may be associated with an ascending aortic aneurysm.
3. Is this a T1W or a T2W image?
4. What is the difference between a true and false aneurysm?

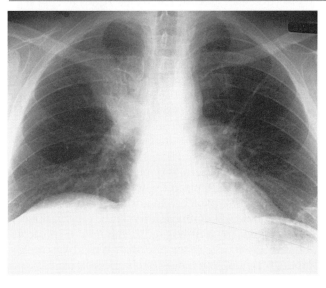
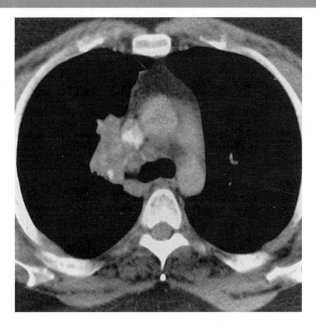

1. Which pulmonary neoplasm is the most likely cause for this centrally obstructing mass that contains calcification?
2. Are carcinoids benign or malignant neoplasms?
3. Name the hormone that carcinoids may secrete ectopically.
4. What percentage of carcinoids demonstrate calcification on CT images?

C A S E 7 3

Ascending Aortic Aneurysm Secondary to Cystic Medial Necrosis

1. Ascending aortic aneurysm.

2. Cystic medial necrosis (Marfan's and Ehlers-Danlos syndromes), atherosclerosis, and syphilis.

3. T1W (note the bright signal intensity of mediastinal fat).

4. A true aneurysm has an intact aortic wall; a false aneurysm is characterized by a disrupted aortic wall.

Reference

Fraser RS, Colman N, Müller NL, Paré PD: Masses situated predominately in the middle-posterior compartment. In: *Fraser and Paré's Diagnosis of Diseases of the Chest*, fourth edition. Philadelphia, WB Saunders, 1999, pp 2951–2955.

Cross-Reference

Thoracic Radiology: THE REQUISITES, pp 447–449.

Comment

The coronal MRI in the figure reveals marked aneurysmal dilation of the ascending aorta. An *aneurysm* is defined as an abnormal dilation of a vessel. With regard to the ascending aorta, there is some variability in diameter with increasing patient age, but a diameter of greater than 4 cm is generally considered abnormal.

Aneurysms may be classified on the basis of the integrity of aorta wall (true vs. false), location, and shape. With regard to shape, fusiform aneurysms are characterized by cylindrical dilation of the entire circumference of the aorta, and saccular aneurysms are characterized by a focal outpouching of the aorta. Fusiform aneurysms are most commonly associated with atherosclerosis, whereas saccular aneurysms are most often mycotic.

Ascending aortic aneurysms are less common than descending thoracic aortic aneurysms. Although aneurysmal dilation of the ascending aorta is frequently caused by atherosclerosis, this process usually involves other portions of the aorta as well. Isolated aneurysmal dilation of the ascending aorta is most closely associated with cystic medial necrosis. This disorder may be idiopathic or associated with connective tissue disorders such as Ehlers-Danlos and Marfan's syndromes. Syphilis, once a relatively common cause of ascending aortic aneurysms, is now rare.

The major complication of aneurysms is rupture. The risk of rupture is related to the size of the aneurysm and significantly increases when the aortic diameter exceeds 6 cm.

Notes

C A S E 7 4

Carcinoid

1. Carcinoid.

2. Malignant.

3. Adrenocorticotropic hormone.

4. Approximately 30%.

Reference

Rosado de Christenson ML, Abbott GF, Kirejczyk WM, Galvin JR, Travis WD: Thoracic carcinoids: radiologic-pathologic correlation. *Radiographics* 19:707–736, 1999.

Cross-Reference

Thoracic Radiology: THE REQUISITES, pp 323–325.

Comment

The frontal chest radiograph demonstrates a central, right hilar mass with associated partial atelectasis of the right upper lobe. The CT image demonstrates a partially calcified right hilar mass that obstructs the right upper lobe bronchus. The imaging features are characteristic of a central carcinoid tumor.

Bronchial carcinoid tumors are uncommon neuroendocrine neoplasms that occur centrally (80%) more commonly than peripherally (20%). Affected patients are usually in the third to seventh decade of life and typically present with cough, hemoptysis, and postobstructive pneumonia.

On chest radiographs, carcinoids typically appear as a central, hilar, or perihilar mass that may be associated with postobstructive atelectasis, pneumonia, mucoid impaction, or bronchiectasis. On CT, carcinoids typically demonstrate well-defined margins and slightly lobulated borders. Carcinoids are usually located close to the central bronchi, usually near airway bifurcations. Calcification is observed in approximately 30% of cases on CT but is not usually evident on conventional radiographs. Most lesions demonstrate intense contrast enhancement.

A minority of carcinoids present as a solitary pulmonary nodule in the periphery of the lung. Typical carcinoid tumors in the periphery of the lungs usually grow at a slow rate. Atypical carcinoids, which comprise 10% of all carcinoids, occur most often in the lung periphery. These lesions are usually large at the time of presentation and grow at a faster rate than typical carcinoids. Although typical carcinoids rarely metastasize, atypical carcinoids exhibit metastases in up to half of patients.

Therapy of carcinoid tumors consists of surgical resection, with a more aggressive surgical approach for atypical lesions. Adjuvant chemotherapy has also been employed with some success in patients with advanced atypical carcinoid tumors. Typical carcinoids have an excellent prognosis, with a 5-year survival of 92%. In contrast, atypical carcinoids are associated with a 5-year survival of 69%.

Notes

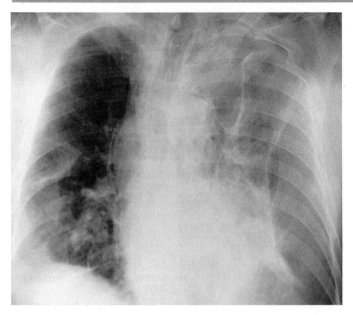

1. Name the syndrome that refers to esophageal perforation due to repeated episodes of vomiting.
2. Name at least three other causes of esophageal perforation.
3. Name two sites of abnormal, extraalveolar air collections that may be associated with esophageal perforation.
4. Are pleural complications of esophageal perforation more commonly left- or right-sided?

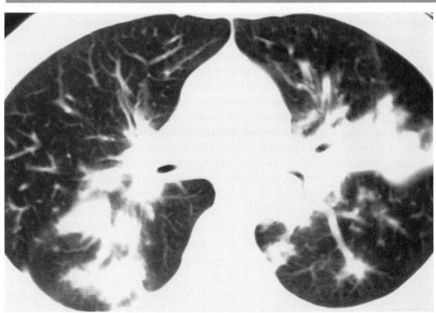

1. In an HIV-positive patient, what is the most likely cause for these CT findings?
2. What organ system is most commonly involved by this neoplasm?
3. Name the demographic group of HIV-positive patients that is most commonly affected by this neoplasm.
4. Is Kaposi's sarcoma (KS) gallium-avid?

Boerhaave's Syndrome

1. Boerhaave's syndrome.

2. Iatrogenic, impacted foreign body, obstructing neoplasm, and trauma.

3. Pneumomediastinum and pneumothorax.

4. Left-sided.

Reference
Gastrointestinal Radiology: THE REQUISITES, p 28.

Cross-Reference
Thoracic Radiology: THE REQUISITES, pp 464–466.

Comment
Esophageal perforation is the most common cause of acute mediastinitis and may occur secondary to a variety of mechanisms. Boerhaave's syndrome refers to transmural perforation of the distal esophagus that occurs secondary to repeated episodes of vomiting.

Patients with esophageal perforation typically present with symptoms of fever, leukocytosis, dysphagia, and retrosternal chest pain, which often radiates into the neck. Pneumomediastinum is a frequent chest radiographic finding, as demonstrated in this case (note the presence of an abnormal lucency surrounding the ascending aorta and aortic arch and extending into the soft tissues of the lower neck). Additional chest radiographic findings may include diffuse mediastinal widening, pneumothorax (note the presence of a left hydropneumothorax in the figure), pleural effusion, and empyema. When the diagnosis of esophageal perforation is delayed, additional complications may include mediastinal abscess, esophagopleural fistula, and esophagobronchial fistula.

A diagnosis of suspected esophageal perforation can be confirmed by performing a fluoroscopic examination of the esophagus following the administration of water-soluble contrast medium. Such a study demonstrates extravasation of contrast at the site of perforation. CT may be helpful to delineate the location and extent of fluid collections in cases that have progressed to mediastinal abscess formation.

It is important to be aware that a delay of more than 24 hours in the diagnosis of this complication is associated with high morbidity and mortality rates. Thus, prompt diagnosis and treatment are critical.

Notes

Kaposi's Sarcoma

1. Kaposi's sarcoma.

2. Skin.

3. Homosexual men.

4. No.

Reference
Staples CA, Müller NL: Thoracic imaging. In: Reeders JWAJ, Matheson JR, Eds: *AIDS Imaging: A Practical Clinical Approach*. London, WB Saunders, 1998, p 150.

Cross-Reference
Thoracic Radiology: THE REQUISITES, pp 145–149.

Comment
KS is the most common AIDS-related neoplasm and occurs predominantly, but not exclusively, in homosexual men. KS is a multicentric neoplasm that arises from endothelial cells. It may involve multiple organ systems, including the skin, lymphatics, lungs, and gastrointestinal system. Interestingly, there is strong evidence to support a pathogenic link between human herpesvirus 8 and KS.

The CT image in this case demonstrates characteristic lung parenchymal abnormalities of KS, including a peribronchovascular distribution of consolidation and poorly defined lung nodules. Less commonly observed lung parenchymal findings may include interlobular septal thickening and ground-glass attenuation. The latter is usually observed around the perimeter of lung nodules and masses. Pleural effusions and thoracic lymph node enlargement are relatively common thoracic manifestations of KS and frequently accompany pulmonary parenchymal abnormalities.

Nuclear medicine imaging may be helpful in the assessment of HIV-positive patients with suspected pulmonary KS. Unlike pulmonary infections and lymphoma, KS is not gallium-avid. Thus, in an HIV-positive patient with diffuse parenchymal abnormalities, the absence of increased gallium activity within the lungs can help confirm the diagnosis of KS and exclude a coexisting infection or alternative diagnosis such as lymphoma.

Notes

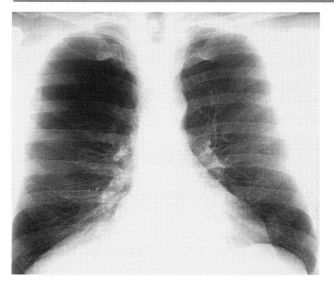
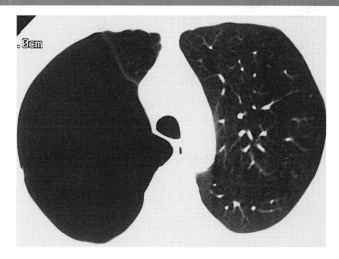

1. Define a bulla.
2. Define a bleb.
3. Name at least two potential complications of bullae.
4. What is the treatment for symptomatic bullae?

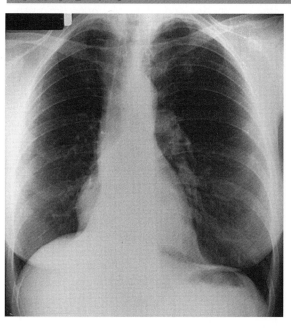
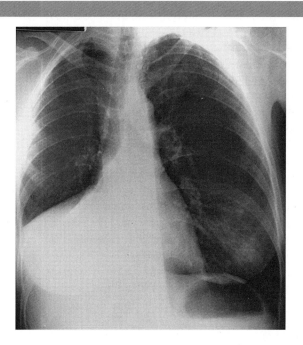

1. What lobe(s) is collapsed in the first figure?
2. What lobe(s) is collapsed in the second figure?
3. In a patient with a known extrathoracic primary neoplasm, what is the likely cause for lobar collapse?
4. Name at least three common sites of primary malignancies that are associated with endobronchial metastases.

C A S E   7 7

Bulla

1. A bulla is a sharply demarcated area of emphysema measuring more than 1 cm in diameter and possessing a well-defined wall less than 1 mm in thickness.

2. A bleb is a gas-containing space within the visceral pleura of the lung.

3. Pneumothorax, infection, and hemorrhage.

4. Surgical resection (bullectomy).

Reference

Wilson AG: Diseases of the airways. In: Armstrong P, Wilson AG, Dee P, Hansell DM, Eds: *Images of Diseases of the Chest*, second edition. St. Louis, Mosby, 1995, pp 856-857.

Cross-Reference

Thoracic Radiology: THE REQUISITES, pp 58-59, 295.

Comment

The chest radiograph and the CT image demonstrate a large bulla within the right upper lobe.

Bullae may develop in association with any type of emphysema, but they are most commonly associated with paraseptal and centrilobular emphysema. However, they are not always associated with diffuse emphysema.

Bullae usually enlarge over months to years, but the growth rate is quite variable. Occasionally, bullae can become quite large and may be focal in distribution. Large bullae may compromise respiratory function. The resulting syndrome has been referred to by various terms, including *bullous emphysema, vanishing lung syndrome*, and *primary bullous disease of the lung*. This entity occurs most often in young men and is characterized by large, progressive upper lobe bullous disease. Although it may occur in nonsmokers, most affected patients are smokers.

CT is the preferred modality for the assessment of patients with suspected bullous emphysema. CT is helpful for delineating the number, size, and location of bullae. It can also assess the degree of compression of underlying normal lung and determine the presence and severity of emphysema in the remaining portion of the lung parenchyma.

In symptomatic patients, surgical resection of bullae can result in marked improvement in pulmonary function. The greatest benefit from surgery is observed in patients with a large bulla (occupying $\geq$ 50% of a hemithorax), a moderate reduction in forced expiratory volume in 1 second (FEV_1), a rapid onset of dyspnea, and no evidence of generalized emphysema.

Notes

C A S E   7 8

Right Middle and Lower Lobe Collapse Secondary to Endobronchial Metastases

1. Right lower lobe.

2. Right middle lobe and right lower lobe.

3. Endobronchial metastases.

4. Kidney, melanoma, thyroid, breast, and colon.

Reference

Fraser RS, Colman N, Müller NL, Paré PD: Pulmonary neoplasms. In: *Fraser and Paré's Diagnosis of Diseases of the Chest*, fourth edition. Philadelphia, WB Saunders, 1999, pp 1397-1399.

Cross-Reference

Thoracic Radiology: THE REQUISITES, pp 35-48, 337.

Comment

The chest radiograph in the first figure demonstrates complete collapse of the right lower lobe. A subsequent radiograph (second figure) performed several weeks later reveals combined collapse of the right middle and lower lobes. In the first figure, note the characteristic triangular opacity in the right retrocardiac region that is bordered by a displaced major fissure. The appearance is similar to that observed in cases of left lower lobe collapse. In the second figure, note the further increase in degree of volume loss, with displacement of minor and major fissures, accompanied by increased opacity that obscures the right hemidiaphragmatic contour. The appearance is typical of combined right middle and lower lobe collapse.

Combined right middle and lower lobe collapse can occur when a tumor obstructs the bronchus intermedius. This combination is much more common than combined right upper and right middle lobe collapse because the bronchi to these lobes are remote from one another. When the latter combination occurs, the appearance is identical to left upper lobe collapse.

In this patient, the combined lobar collapse occurred secondary to endobronchial metastatic disease. Also note the presence of pulmonary metastases, best visualized in the left lung. Endobronchial metastases are uncommon and are found in less than 5% of patients at autopsy. Presenting symptoms may include cough, wheeze, and hemoptysis. Coughing may infrequently result in expectoration of tumor fragments; rarely, this is the first indication of metastatic disease.

Radiographic findings in the setting of partial airway obstruction include oligemia and air trapping. In the setting of complete bronchial obstruction, findings include lobar, segmental, or subsegmental atelectasis and postobstructive pneumonitis. A hilar or central mass may also be evident.

Notes

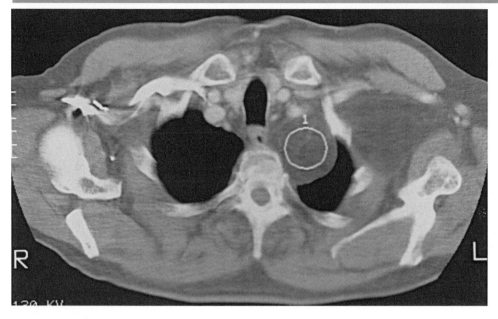

1. A region-of-interest measurement of this mass demonstrated Hounsfield units consistent with fat attenuation. What are the two most likely diagnoses?

2. How can you explain the spread of this mass into the axilla?

3. Although this mass is predominantly fat attenuation, it contains a few strands of soft tissue attenuation. Does the latter finding exclude the diagnosis of lipoma?

4. What feature of this mass favors a benign diagnosis?

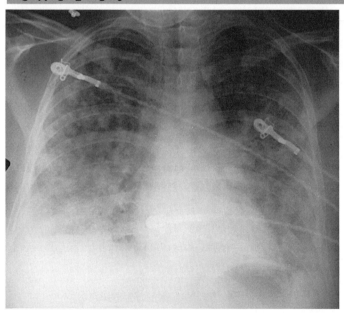

1. Which type of viral pneumonia typically presents with a diffuse distribution of poorly defined lung nodules?

2. What is the approximate overall incidence of pneumonia in patients with chickenpox?

3. Do pregnant women have a higher or lower incidence of varicella pneumonia than the general population?

4. What is the typical radiographic appearance of healed varicella pneumonia?

Lipoma

1. Lipoma and liposarcoma.

2. The mass is likely extrapleural in location rather than truly mediastinal and probably spreads over the apex of the lung into the left axilla.

3. No.

4. Pliability/lack of invasiveness.

Reference

Pugatch R, Spirn PW: Mediastinal neoplasms. In: Taveras JM, Ferrucci JT, Eds: *Radiology: Diagnosis, Imaging, Intervention*, Volume I. Philadelphia, Lippincott-Raven, 1998, 76:1–10 (looseleaf).

Cross-Reference

None.

Comment

The CT image demonstrates a fat attenuation mass that contains several strands of soft tissue attenuation. The mass extends into the left axilla, but there is no invasion of the ribs or vessels.

Lipomas may occur in a variety of locations in the thorax, including the mediastinum, chest wall, extrapleural space, esophagus, heart, airway, and, rarely, the lung parenchyma. Although lipomas typically appear as well-marginated lesions characterized by homogeneous fat attenuation, soft tissue elements may be observed. In such cases, it may not be possible to distinguish lipoma from thymolipoma or low-grade liposarcoma. The pliability and lack of invasiveness of lipomas may aid in their differentiation from liposarcomas; for example, lipomas typically drape around adjacent vessels, ribs, and mediastinal structures without invading them. In contrast with lipomas, liposarcomas typically contain a larger soft tissue component, have irregular margins, and frequently invade adjacent mediastinal and chest wall structures. Thus, the presence of well-defined margins and lack of invasiveness favor a diagnosis of lipoma over liposarcoma. The diagnosis of lipoma was confirmed at pathology.

Notes

Varicella-Zoster (Chickenpox)

1. Varicella-zoster (chickenpox).

2. Roughly 15%.

3. Higher.

4. Diffuse, discrete pulmonary calcifications.

Reference

Fraser RS, Colman N, Müller NL, Paré PD: Viruses, mycoplasmas, chlamydiae, and rickettsiae. In: *Fraser and Paré's Diagnosis and Diseases of the Chest*, fourth edition. Philadelphia, WB Saunders, 1999, pp 999–1004.

Cross-Reference

Thoracic Radiology: THE REQUISITES, p 113.

Comment

The chest radiograph demonstrates a diffuse distribution of poorly defined small lung nodules, some of which have coalesced to form areas of consolidation. The appearance is typical of varicella-zoster (chickenpox) pneumonia.

The varicella-zoster virus is seen in two clinical forms: chickenpox (varicella) and zoster (shingles). Chickenpox represents the primary form of the virus and usually presents as disseminated disease in previously uninfected individuals. On the other hand, zoster represents reactivation of a latent virus and typically manifests as a unilateral dermatologic skin eruption. Although either form of the virus may be associated with pneumonia, the majority of cases occur in association with chickenpox.

The overall incidence of pneumonia in patients with chickenpox is approximately 15%. Predisposing factors include leukemia, lymphoma, immunodeficiency, and pregnancy. Both the incidence and severity of varicella pneumonia are significantly higher in pregnant women than in the general population.

Acute chickenpox pneumonia is most common in adult patients with severe cutaneous disease. Affected patients typically present 2 or 3 days following the appearance of a skin eruption with symptoms of cough, dyspnea, tachypnea, and pleuritic chest pain.

Acute chickenpox pneumonia is associated with a mortality rate as high as 10%. In patients who survive the infection, clinical improvement usually precedes radiographic clearing by several weeks. A characteristic radiologic finding in patients with healed varicella pneumonia is the presence of diffuse discrete pulmonary calcifications.

Notes

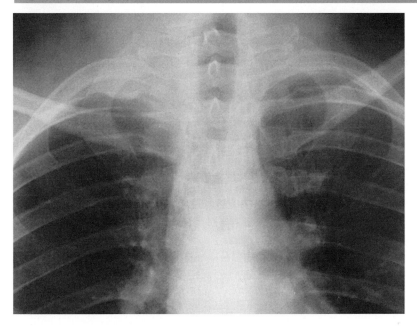

1. Name at least four causes of a unilateral, enlarged apical cap.

2. What is the term used to describe a bronchogenic carcinoma that arises at the apex of the lung?

3. Regarding extrapleural apical lesions, are their margins usually smooth or irregular?

4. This patient presented with a palpable right-sided neck mass. Name two possible causes for the enlarged apical cap in this case.

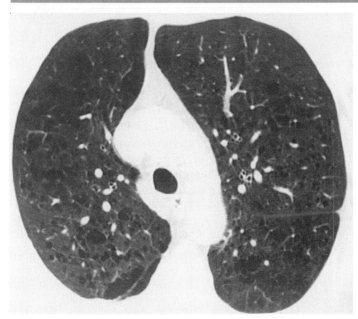

1. What is the etiology of the abnormal low-attenuation areas present in both lungs on this HRCT image?

2. What types of emphysema are evident in this case?

3. What type of emphysema is most closely associated with cigarette smoking?

4. What portion of the lungs is most commonly affected by this type of emphysema?

CASE 81

Apical Cap Secondary to Extrapleural Abscess Extending From the Neck

1. Bronchogenic carcinoma, lymphoma extending from the neck or mediastinum, extrapleural hematoma related to injury, extrapleural abscess extending from the neck, and radiation fibrosis.

2. Superior sulcus tumor.

3. Smooth.

4. Extrapleural extension of neck abscess and lymphoma.

Reference

McLoud TC, Isler RJ, Novelline RA, et al: The apical cap. *AJR Am J Roentgenol* 137:299–306, 1981.

Cross-Reference

None.

Comment

The term *apical cap* has been used to describe the presence of an opacity located in the extreme apex of the lung on chest radiographs. On chest radiographs of normal, asymptomatic patients, you will often observe the apical cap as an irregular opacity located over the apex of the lung, usually measuring less than 5 mm in diameter. The lower margin is usually sharply marginated but often demonstrates an undulating border. Apical caps are thought to represent the result of nonspecific subpleural scarring and apical pleural thickening, and they are usually of no clinical significance. The prevalence of apical caps increases with age.

There are a variety of entities that may result in an enlarged apical cap. The various causes of a unilateral enlarged cap have been listed in Answer 1. With regard to bilaterally enlarged apical caps, they may be associated with radiation fibrosis (e.g., for Hodgkin's disease), mediastinal lipomatosis, and vascular abnormalities such as coarctation of the aorta.

In this case, the presence of a smoothly marginated enlarged right apical cap is due to extension of a neck abscess into the lung apex. Because of the continuity of the fascial planes of the neck with the thoracic apical region, infectious processes originating in the neck may extend into the area of the lung apex, within the extrapleural space. The apical cap in such cases is smoothly marginated, reflecting the extrapleural location. Lymphoma is an additional important consideration in this case. In patients with lymphoma, an apical cap may be produced by extension of lymphadenopathy from the neck or by enlargement of lymph nodes along the apical pleura.

Notes

CASE 82

Emphysema

1. Emphysema.

2. Centrilobular and paraseptal.

3. Centrilobular.

4. Upper lobes.

Reference

Kazerooni EA, Whyte RI, Flint A, Martinez FJ: Imaging of emphysema and lung volume reduction surgery. *Radiographics* 17:1023–1036, 1997.

Cross-Reference

Thoracic Radiology: THE REQUISITES, pp 287–295.

Comment

The HRCT image demonstrates multiple foci of low attenuation, consistent with emphysema. Note the absence of definable walls for most of the areas of abnormal low attenuation.

Features of both centrilobular and paraseptal emphysema are present. Centrilobular emphysema is characterized by multiple small, round foci of abnormally low attenuation without visible walls that are scattered throughout the lung parenchyma. Paraseptal emphysema is characterized by its location within the subpleural regions and adjacent to the interlobar fissures. Foci of paraseptal emphysema often have thin visible walls which correspond to interlobular septa. In this case, paraseptal emphysema is best demonstrated adjacent to the right major fissure and adjacent to the anterior mediastinal pleural surfaces. When larger than a centimeter in size, foci of paraseptal emphysema are most appropriately referred to as "bullae."

HRCT of the chest is highly sensitive and specific for the diagnosis of emphysema. It is particularly helpful for assessing the severity and distribution of emphysema in patients who are potential candidates for lung volume reduction surgery (LVRS). LVRS is a procedure that involves the resection of "target areas" of severely emphysematous lung. Such regions contribute little to pulmonary function and negatively alter respiratory mechanics. LVRS usually involves bilateral wedge resection procedures performed via a median sternotomy.

Improved pulmonary function following LVRS is thought to be due to several factors, including improved elastic recoil of the lungs, correction of ventilation-perfusion mismatches, and improved mechanics of breathing. Patients are selected for the procedure based on a variety of clinical and imaging parameters. With regard to imaging features, preliminary data suggest that patients with a heterogeneous distribution of emphysema with an upper lobe predominance are most likely to benefit from this procedure.

Notes

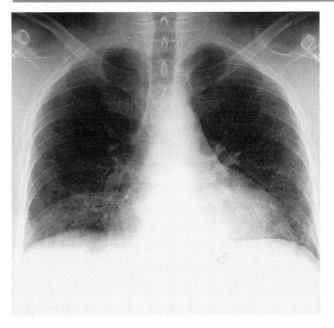

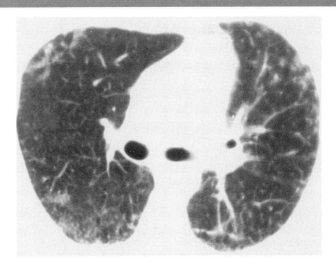

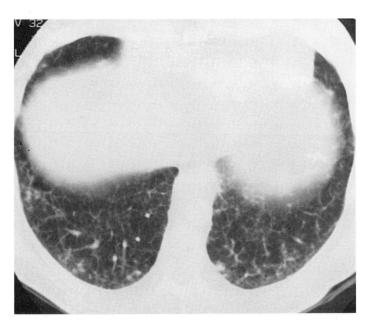

1. This patient has a history of lymphoma and is being treated with bleomycin. What is the most likely cause for the interstitial opacities observed in the first and second figures?

2. Approximately what percentage of patients receiving bleomycin develop pulmonary toxicity?

3. Does simultaneous chest radiation therapy increase or decrease the risk of bleomycin pulmonary toxicity?

4. Would you expect this patient's diffusing capacity (DLCO) to be increased or decreased?

Bleomycin Drug Toxicity

1. Bleomycin pulmonary toxicity.

2. Approximately 4%.

3. Increase.

4. Decreased.

Reference
Aronchick JM, Gefter WB: Drug-induced pulmonary disorders. *Semin Roentgenol* 30:18–34, 1995.

Cross-Reference
Thoracic Radiology: THE REQUISITES, pp 275, 276, 279.

Comment
The chest radiograph in the first figure reveals the presence of reticular opacities within the peripheral and basilar portions of the lung parenchyma. The CT images in the second and third figures demonstrate thickened septal lines, irregular linear opacities, ground-glass opacities, and several tiny lung nodules in a subpleural and basilar predominance.

Bleomycin is an antitumor agent that is used to treat lymphomas, testicular carcinomas, and certain squamous cell carcinomas. Pulmonary toxicity occurs in approximately 4% of patients and is the principal dose-limiting factor for this agent. Pulmonary fibrosis is the most serious pulmonary complication, but an acute hypersensitivity reaction occurs rarely.

Affected patients typically present with an insidious onset of dyspnea, nonproductive cough, and occasional fever. Pulmonary function tests reveal a decreased D_{LCO}, a sensitive measure for early bleomycin lung injury.

Chest radiographs may be normal or may demonstrate reticular opacities in a basilar and subpleural distribution, similar to those observed in idiopathic pulmonary fibrosis. CT is more sensitive that conventional radiographs for detecting interstitial abnormalities and may reveal characteristic findings even when the chest radiograph is normal.

Early detection is important because prompt discontinuation of bleomycin may result in improved pulmonary function and healing of pulmonary damage in patients with early stages of disease. In patients with more advanced disease, the prognosis is variable. Although some patients respond to steroids, others develop progressive fibrosis that may lead to respiratory failure and death.

Notes

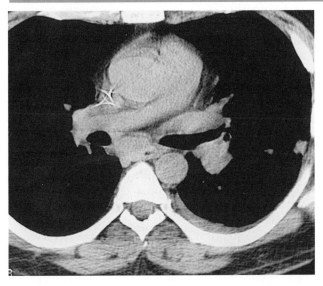

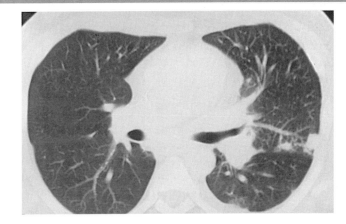

1. In an HIV-positive patient, which fungal infection is most likely to present with pulmonary nodules, pleural effusion, and lymph node enlargement?

2. Are pleural effusions and thoracic lymph node enlargement more commonly observed in immunocompetent or immunosuppressed patients with cryptococcal pulmonary infection?

3. What organ system is most commonly affected by this organism?

4. What other organ systems are commonly involved in disseminated cryptococcal infection?

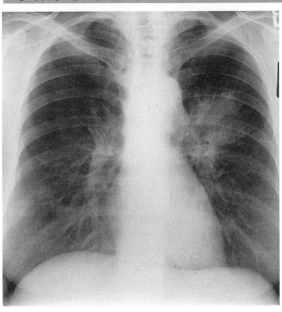

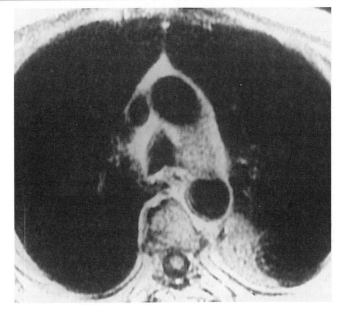

1. Transthoracic biopsy of the lung mass shown in the figures revealed non-small cell lung cancer (NSCLC). Is the presence of an enlarged aortopulmonary window lymph node sufficient proof of metastatic nodal disease?

2. Based on the TNM classification system for NSCLC, if this node is proven malignant, what would be the N status of the patient?

3. Does this nodal status preclude surgical resection?

4. What is the significance of contralateral nodal disease in patients with NSCLC?

Acquired Immunodeficiency Syndrome Cryptococcal Infection

1. *Cryptococcus*.

2. Immunosuppressed.

3. Central nervous system (meningitis).

4. Bone and skin.

Reference

Connolly JE, McAdams HP, Erasmus J, Rosado-de-Christenson ML: Opportunistic fungal pneumonia. *J Thoracic Imaging* 14:51–62, 1999.

Cross-Reference

Thoracic Radiology: THE REQUISITES, pp 142–145.

Comment

The CT images in this case demonstrate several small pulmonary nodules with associated left hilar and subcarinal lymph node enlargement and a small left pleural effusion. There are a variety of causes of lung nodules in patients with AIDS, including infectious etiologies (fungal, mycobacterial, septic infarcts) and neoplasms (Kaposi's sarcoma, lymphoma).

Prior to the AIDS epidemic and the advent of immunosuppressive therapies, most cryptococcal infections occurred in immunocompetent hosts. It is estimated that roughly 70% of such infections now occur in immunosuppressed patients. In immunocompetent hosts, the infection is usually localized to the lung. In contrast, in immunosuppressed patients, dissemination to the central nervous system and skin is common. Pulmonary symptoms are uncommon in both groups. However, immunosuppressed patients with disseminated disease frequently present with symptoms related to the central nervous system or skeletal system.

There are a variety of imaging features associated with this infection. Common manifestations in both immunosuppressed and immunocompetent hosts include solitary or multiple pulmonary nodules and masses and segmental or lobar consolidation. Other features, including diffuse reticulonodular opacities, cavitating nodules or masses, pleural effusion, and mediastinal and hilar lymph node enlargement, are more commonly observed in immunosuppressed patients than in normal hosts.

Notes

Bronchogenic Carcinoma With N2 Nodal Disease

1. No.

2. N2.

3. No.

4. It precludes surgical resection.

Reference

Boiselle PM, Patz EF, Vining DJ, et al: Imaging of mediastinal lymph nodes: CT, MR, and FDG PET. *Radiographics* 18:1061–1069, 1998.

Cross-Reference

Thoracic Radiology: THE REQUISITES, pp 316–323.

Comment

In patients with NSCLC, the nodal status provides important information for determining prognosis and planning appropriate therapy. According to the TNM classification system, nodal involvement is graded from N0 to N3 as follows:

N0 = no demonstrable metastases to regional lymph nodes

N1 = metastasis to lymph nodes in the peribronchial region, the ipsilateral hilar region, or both, including direct extension

N2 = metastasis to ipsilateral mediastinal nodes and subcarinal nodes

N3 = metastasis to contralateral mediastinal or hilar nodes, ipsilateral or contralateral scalene or supraclavicular nodes

CT and MRI play an important but limited role in the assessment of nodal status in patients with bronchogenic carcinoma. These imaging modalities rely primarily on anatomic features of lymph nodes, most notably lymph node size (short axis >1 cm diameter is generally considered abnormal). This strategy is associated with sensitivities in the range of 60% to 79% and specificities in the range of 60% to 80%. Thus, for staging purposes, enlarged nodes must be evaluated by biopsy. The primary role of these modalities is to identify the location of enlarged nodes. This information allows appropriate biopsy procedures to be planned.

In recent years, 2-[fluorine-18]fluoro-2-deoxy-D-glucose (FDG) positron emission tomography (PET) imaging has been shown to be superior to CT and MRI in the assessment of mediastinal lymph nodes. This technique relies on physiologic (glucose metabolism) rather than anatomic features to identify abnormal lymph nodes. Thus, it has the potential to identify neoplastic involvement within small nodes and to differentiate enlarged, hyperplastic nodes from neoplastic nodes.

Notes

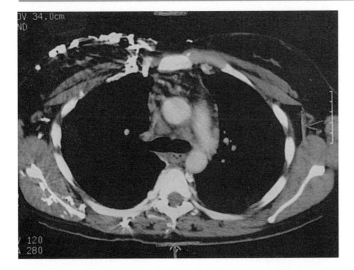

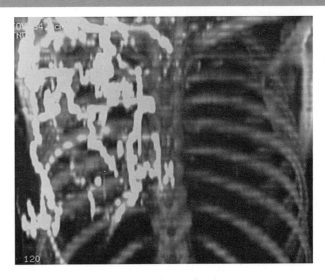

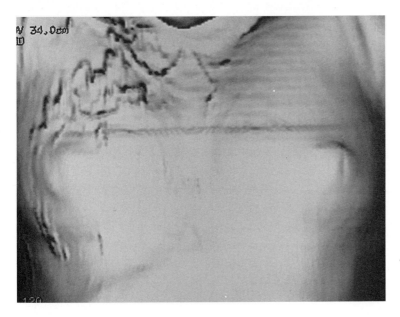

1. What is the most common cause of superior vena cava (SVC) syndrome?

2. Name at least one common benign cause of SVC syndrome.

3. What do the enhancing serpiginous structures in the right chest wall represent?

4. What are the typical clinical symptoms of a patient with SVC obstruction?

Superior Vena Cava Syndrome

1. Malignancy—bronchogenic carcinoma.

2. Long-term intravenous devices; fibrosing mediastinitis.

3. Chest wall collateral vessels.

4. Edema of the face, neck, upper extremities and thorax; headache; visual disturbances; and reduced level of consciousness.

Reference

Fraser RS, Colman N, Müller NL, Paré PD: Mediastinal disease. In: *Fraser and Paré's Diagnosis of Diseases of the Chest*, fourth edition. Philadelphia, WB Saunders, 1999, pp 2949–2950.

Cross-Reference

Thoracic Radiology: THE REQUISITES, pp 466–467, 470, 471.

Comment

The SVC syndrome is caused by obstruction of the SVC by either external compression, intraluminal thrombosis, neoplastic infiltration, or a combination of these processes. The vast majority of cases occur secondary to a neoplastic process, most commonly bronchogenic carcinoma (especially small cell carcinoma). Lymphoma and metastatic carcinoma are additional malignant causes. There are a variety of benign etiologies, including long-term intravenous devices (e.g., Hickman catheters and permanent pacemakers) and fibrosing mediastinitis (e.g., histoplasmosis).

Chest radiographs frequently demonstrate a mass in the right paratracheal region, which may be accompanied by distention of the azygos vein. In the setting of fibrosing mediastinitis, the right paratracheal mass is frequently calcified. In patients who develop thrombosis of the SVC due to an indwelling catheter, lateral displacement of the catheter may be seen. The diagnosis of SVC obstruction can be confirmed by CT, MRI, or conventional venography. On CT, the diagnosis is based on decreased or absent contrast opacification of the SVC in conjunction with opacification of collateral vessels. Both findings are necessary to make a reliable diagnosis.

In the first figure, note the presence of extensive venous collateral vessels, which are most prominent in the right anterior chest wall. These vessels are seen to a better degree on the coronal 3D reconstruction image in the second figure. Also note the prominent dilated chest wall veins on the shaded surface display image in the third figure, which demonstrates the external visibility of these vessels.

When you observe collateral venous vessels, you should always search for a central venous obstruction. In the first figure, note the poorly opacified SVC that is partially compressed by an adjacent enlarged lymph node. Below this level, the SVC was completely occluded.

Notes

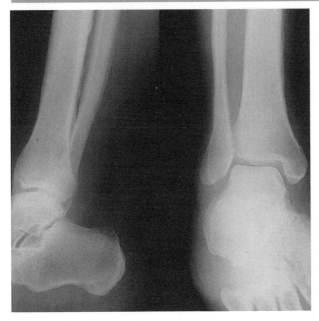
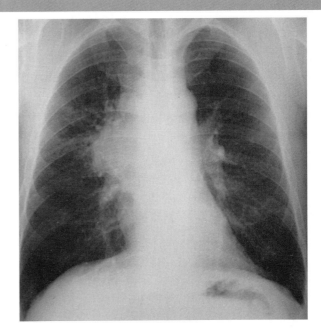

1. What is the term used to describe the presence of periosteal reaction in association with pulmonary disease?

2. Are benign or malignant disorders more commonly associated with this process?

3. When this process occurs in association with a pulmonary malignancy, what is the usual response of the periosteal reaction following pulmonary neoplasm resection?

4. Is this skeletal process typically symptomatic?

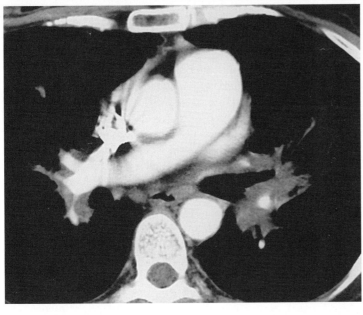
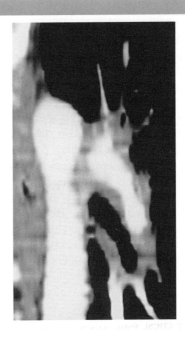

1. Does this patient have an acute pulmonary embolus?

2. What is the cause of the focal decrease in caliber of the descending left pulmonary artery?

3. In patients with sarcoidosis, how frequently do enlarged nodes result in compression of pulmonary arteries?

4. What vascular structure appears abnormally dilated in the first figure?

CASE 87

Hypertrophic Pulmonary Osteoarthropathy

1. Hypertrophic pulmonary osteoarthropathy (HPOA).

2. Malignant.

3. Resolution.

4. Yes—it is usually associated with pain, swelling, and stiffness.

Reference

Fraser RS, Colman, N, Müller NL, Paré PD: Investigative methods in chest disease. In: *Fraser and Paré's Diagnosis of Diseases of the Chest*, fourth edition. Philadelphia, WB Saunders, 1999, pp 396-397.

Cross-Reference

Thoracic Radiology: THE REQUISITES, pp 502-503.

Comment

The radiographs of the right ankle shown in the first figure reveal the presence of smoothly marginated periosteal reaction along the shafts of the distal tibia and fibula. A similar appearance was present in radiographs of the remaining extremities (not shown).

The term *HPOA* is used to describe the association between this skeletal condition and visceral disease within an organ supplied by the vagal or glossopharyngeal nerves. Although there are a variety of pulmonary and extrapulmonary causes of this condition, malignant pulmonary neoplasms account for the vast majority (90%) of cases. Because of this strong association, you should always recommend that a patient with evidence of HPOA undergo a chest radiograph to assess for pulmonary neoplasm or other causes of pulmonary disease. Note the large central neoplasm on the chest radiograph of this patient in the second figure. Common nonneoplastic pulmonary conditions include cystic fibrosis and idiopathic pulmonary fibrosis. Localized fibrous lesions of the pleura are also frequently associated with this condition.

The underlying mechanism of this condition is poorly understood, but it probably occurs due to increased blood flow secondary to an abnormal neurohormonal reflex arc. Interestingly, following resection of an associated thoracic malignancy, this process usually disappears.

Notes

CASE 88

Extrinsic Compression of Pulmonary Arteries (Sarcoid)

1. No.

2. Extrinsic compression by adjacent nodal tissue.

3. Rarely.

4. Main pulmonary artery.

Reference

Fraser RS, Colman N, Müller NL, Paré PD: Sarcoidosis. In: *Fraser and Paré's Diagnosis of Diseases of the Chest*, fourth edition. Philadelphia, WB Saunders, 1999, pp 1545-1550.

Cross-Reference

Thoracic Radiology: THE REQUISITES, pp 415-417.

Comment

The CT pulmonary angiogram images in the first (axial) and second (coronal reformation) figures reveal narrowing of the descending left pulmonary artery and superior segment right lower lobe pulmonary artery by adjacent nodal tissue.

This patient has a history of sarcoidosis. Occasionally, enlarged nodes in patients with sarcoidosis are sufficiently large to compress the bronchi. Rarely, enlarged nodes may result in narrowing of pulmonary arteries, as demonstrated in this case. Massively enlarged right paratracheal nodes have been reported to obstruct the superior vena cava.

When interpreting CT pulmonary angiograms, it is important to distinguish pulmonary emboli from extrinsic abnormalities such as lymph nodes. Note the absence of intrinsic filling defects within the pulmonary vasculature in this case. One additional distinguishing feature is the size of the pulmonary arteries. In the setting of an acute pulmonary embolus, the affected vessel is often dilated. In contrast, when extrinsically compressed, the vessel will be abnormally narrowed. Extrinsic compression may be more difficult to distinguish from chronic pulmonary emboli, which result in mural rather than central pulmonary artery filling defects. Recognition that the abnormal soft tissue attenuation material is extrinsic rather than intrinsic to the vessel allows one to exclude chronic pulmonary embolus. Although this distinction can usually be made readily on conventional axial images (as is true in this case), supplemental multiplanar reformatted images are helpful for difficult cases.

Notes

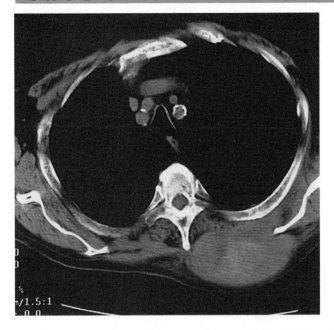 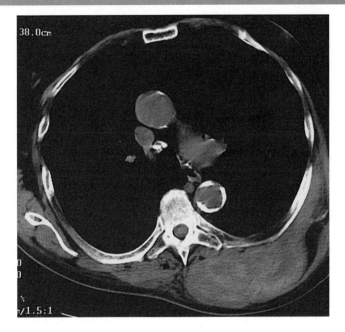

1. This patient has a history of hemophilia. What is the likely cause for this posterior chest wall mass?
2. What does the high-attenuation component of the mass represent on this unenhanced CT scan study?
3. Name at least two potential complications of intramuscular hemorrhage.
4. How is hemophilia genetically transmitted?

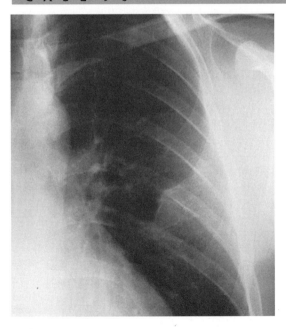 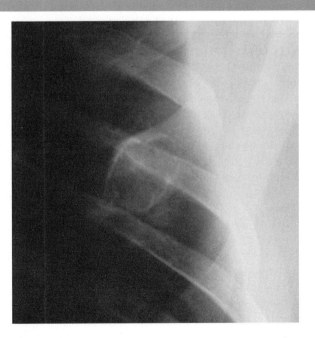

1. What feature suggests a benign, nonaggressive etiology of this rib lesion?
2. Name at least two likely causes of this rib lesion.
3. Name an entity that may be associated with chronic infiltrative lung disease and lucent bone lesions.
4. Name at least three primary neoplasms that are frequently associated with lytic bone metastases.

C A S E 8 9

Chest Wall Hematoma in Hemophilia

1. Hematoma.

2. Acute hemorrhage.

3. Joint contractures, ischemic myopathy, neuropathy, pressure necrosis of adjacent bone, and pseudotumor formation.

4. X-linked recessive; thus, hemophilia is transmitted by females but primarily affects males.

Reference

Hermann G, Gilbert MS, Abdelwahab F: Hemophilia: evaluation of musculoskeletal involvement with CT, sonography, and MR imaging. *AJR Am J Roentgenol* 158:119–123, 1992.

Cross-Reference

None.

Comment

The CT images reveal a large, well-marginated, heterogeneous posterior chest wall mass with its epicenter in the left paraspinal musculature. The high attenuation of this mass on an unenhanced CT is consistent with the diagnosis of acute intramuscular hematoma, a known complication of hemophilia.

Hemophilia refers to a disorder characterized by a coagulation defect caused by a deficiency of clotting factor. Repetitive bleeding into the musculoskeletal system is the most common complication of this condition. The joint spaces are the most common site of spontaneous bleeding. Hemarthrosis is frequently complicated by arthritis. The soft tissues, particularly large muscle groups, are also a relatively common site of hemorrhage. The most commonly affected muscle groups are the iliopsoas, quadriceps, and gastrocnemius. If bleeding into the hematoma is replaced by fibrous tissue, a permanent contracture may develop. Encapsulation of a hematoma may result in the formation of a pseudotumor.

Cross-sectional imaging studies can be helpful for identifying the site and extent of intramuscular hematomas in patients with hemophilia. Because of its relative low cost and lack of ionizing radiation, ultrasonography is usually the preferred modality for this purpose. In patients with large hematomas, CT and MRI are occasionally helpful for determining the extent of hemorrhage, estimating the age of hemorrhage, and demonstrating the effect of the hemorrhage on adjacent organs.

Notes

C A S E 9 0

Enchondroma

1. Well-circumscribed, sclerotic margins.

2. Fibrous dysplasia, aneurysmal bone cyst, enchondroma, nonossifying fibroma, and histiocytosis X.

3. Histiocytosis X (although pulmonary involvement is usually not accompanied by bone lesions).

4. Lung, breast (lytic or blastic), kidney, and thyroid.

Reference

Fraser RS, Colman N, Müller NL, Paré PD: The chest wall. In: *Fraser and Paré's Diagnosis of Diseases of the Chest,* fourth edition. Philadelphia, WB Saunders, 1999, p 3031.

Cross-Reference

None.

Comment

The coned-down chest radiograph in the first figure and the coned-down rib radiograph in the second figure reveal a well-circumscribed, expansile, lucent lesion in the left fourth anterior rib with sclerotic margins. The well-defined, sclerotic margins suggest a nonaggressive rather than aggressive (e.g., neoplasm, infection) etiology. In contrast, aggressive lucent lesions are typically characterized by poorly defined margins.

There are a variety of causes of benign lucent rib lesions. Careful inspection of this lesion reveals subtle foci of calcification within the lucent center of this lesion. This finding suggests a cartilaginous lesion such as enchondroma. In roughly 50% of cases, such lesions demonstrate calcification, which is usually manifested by punctate foci or rings and arcs of calcification. Enchondromas are asymptomatic unless complicated by pathologic fracture or rare malignant degeneration to chondrosarcoma. The latter should be suspected when a patient with an enchondroma presents with pain in the absence of trauma.

The most common nonneoplastic lesion of the thoracic skeleton is fibrous dysplasia. In patients with this disorder, the rib lesion is usually monostotic and asymptomatic. However, patients may present with symptoms if the lesion is complicated by pathologic fracture. In cases of polyostotic fibrous dysplasia, there is usually a unilateral predominance. Rarely, the degree of thoracic involvement is sufficient to result in progressive restrictive lung disease, pulmonary hypertension, and cor pulmonale. McCune-Albright syndrome refers to the presence of polyostotic fibrous dysplasia accompanied by café au lait skin lesions and precocious puberty.

Notes

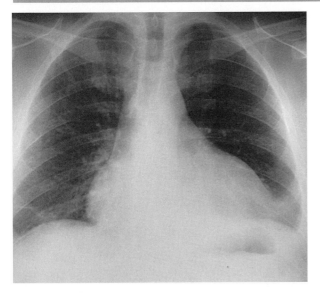
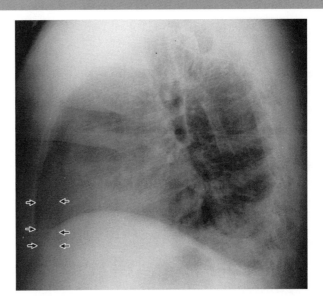

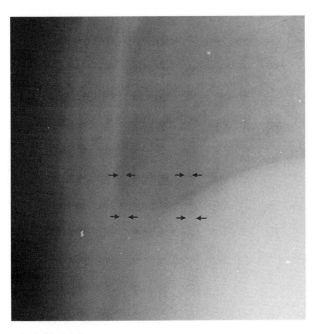

1. What structure is delineated between the *arrows* on the lateral chest radiograph in the second figure?

2. Is this abnormally widened?

3. What do the lucencies on either side of this structure represent?

4. What descriptor is used to characterize the typical appearance of the cardiac contour in the setting of a pericardial effusion?

Pericardial Effusion

1. Pericardium.

2. Yes—it is widened by the presence of pericardial effusion.

3. Fat.

4. Water bottle.

Reference
Cardiac Radiology: THE REQUISITES, pp 265–270.

Cross-Reference
None.

Comment
The chest radiograph in the first figure demonstrates an enlarged cardiac contour, with a globular configuration. The lateral radiograph in the second figure demonstrates a positive epicardial fat pad sign (EFPS), also referred to as the double-lucency sign. This sign refers to widening (>4 mm) of the soft tissue opacity of the pericardium between the lucent stripes *(arrows)* that represent fat located anterior and posterior (epicardial) to the pericardium. These lucent stripes are demarcated by *paired arrows* on the coned-down image of the lateral chest radiograph in the third figure. The EFPS has a relatively low sensitivity but a high specificity for detecting pericardial effusion.

Chest radiography is associated with a relatively poor sensitivity for detecting pericardial effusions. It has been estimated that roughly 200 ml of pericardial fluid must be present to reliably make the diagnosis radiographically. In contrast, echocardiography is highly sensitive for detecting pericardial effusion and is the study of choice for screening patients with suspected pericardial effusion. MRI may be helpful for characterizing complex pericardial fluid collections.

There are a variety of causes of pericardial effusion, including infection, trauma, radiation therapy, collagen vascular diseases, metabolic disorders, and neoplasms. The most common cause is myocardial infarction with left ventricular failure. Dressler's syndrome refers to the development of pericardial and pleural effusions 2 to 10 weeks following myocardial infarction. Such effusions can be hemorrhagic, particularly in patients who have received anticoagulation therapy. The patient in this case developed pericardial and pleural effusions following myocardial infarction.

Notes

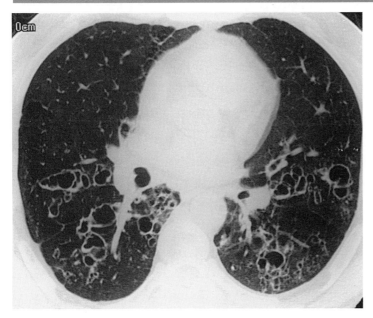

1. Is this a case of cystic lung disease or bronchiectasis?
2. How can you make this distinction?
3. What are the three classifications of bronchiectasis (Reid classification)?
4. Name at least three congenital or developmental disorders associated with bronchiectasis.

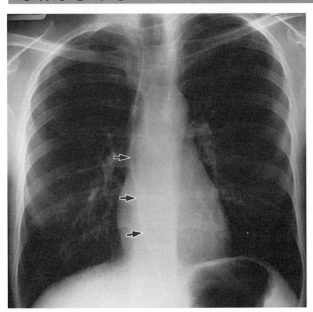

1. Name the structure that is likely responsible for displacement of the azygoesophageal contour *(arrows)* in this patient.
2. Why does this appear as a stripe rather than an interface?
3. What imaging study would be most helpful for further evaluation of this finding?
4. Name at least two causes of thoracic esophageal dysmotility.

Bronchiectasis

1. Bronchiectasis.

2. Many of the cystic spaces are connected, several run parallel to adjacent vessels ("signet-ring sign"), and several have air-fluid levels.

3. Cylindrical, varicose, and cystic (saccular).

4. Williams-Campbell syndrome, cystic fibrosis, primary hypogammaglobulinemia, "yellow nail" syndrome, immotile cilia syndrome (Kartagener's syndrome), Young's syndrome, and Mounier-Kuhn syndrome.

Reference

Shepard JO: The bronchi: an imaging perspective. *J Thorac Imaging* 10:236–254, 1995.

Cross-Reference

Thoracic Radiology: THE REQUISITES, pp 386–391.

Comment

The term *bronchiectasis* refers to abnormal, irreversible dilation of the bronchi. The definitive pathologic description of bronchiectasis was reported by Reid and is based on the morphology of the bronchi and the number of bronchial subdivisions that are present. In cylindrical bronchiectasis, the bronchi are minimally dilated and have a straight, regular contour. The average number of bronchial subdivisions from the hilum to the lung periphery is 16 (17 to 20 is normal). In varicose bronchiectasis, the bronchi demonstrate a beaded appearance with sequential dilation and constriction. The average number of bronchial divisions is 8. In cystic bronchiectasis, the bronchi have a ballooned appearance. The average number of bronchial divisions is only 4.

You can distinguish bronchiectasis from cystic lung disease by using the following criteria. First, when dilated bronchi course perpendicular to the scanning plane, you will always see a pulmonary artery running adjacent to it (signet-ring sign). In contrast, true lung cysts, such as those associated with LAM, are located randomly in the lung parenchyma. Second, when dilated bronchi course parallel to the scanning plane, you will observe that the cystic spaces connect with one another. This feature is nicely demonstrated in this case. Finally, cystic bronchiectasis is often associated with fluid levels, a finding that is not generally observed in cystic lung disease.

Notes

Esophageal Dysmotility (Achalasia)

1. Esophagus.

2. The esophagus is distended with air.

3. Barium swallow.

4. Scleroderma, achalasia, Chagas' disease, systemic diseases (e.g., amyloidosis), and drugs (e.g., anticholinergics).

Reference

Gastrointestinal Radiology: THE REQUISITES, pp 14–16.

Cross-Reference

Thoracic Radiology: THE REQUISITES, pp 424–425, 455–457, 459.

Comment

The azygoesophageal interface is produced by the juxtaposition of aerated lung in the right lower lobe and the soft tissue opacity of the right lateral margin of the azygos vein and/or esophagus. On normal chest radiographs, you will observe the azygoesophageal interface beginning at the level of the azygos arch and extending inferiorly to the level of the diaphragm. It normally produces a concave slope as it curves slightly toward the left. Abnormalities of either the azygos vein (e.g., azygos continuation of the inferior vena cava) or esophagus (e.g., achalasia) may result in rightward displacement of this interface. Subcarinal masses such as bronchogenic cysts and lymph node enlargement may also result in focal rightward displacement of the azygoesophageal interface, usually producing a rightward convexity in the subcarinal region.

The chest radiograph reveals diffuse, rightward displacement of the azygoesophageal contour, which appears as a stripe rather than an interface. When the azygoesophageal contour is displaced by an air-filled, distended esophagus, you will observe a stripe rather than an interface. This patient has a history of achalasia. In most patients with this disorder, the esophagus contains a large amount of retained secretions. Therefore, you will usually see a displaced azygoesophageal interface rather than a stripe. Retained secretions may also result in a discrete air-fluid level within the distended esophagus.

Notes

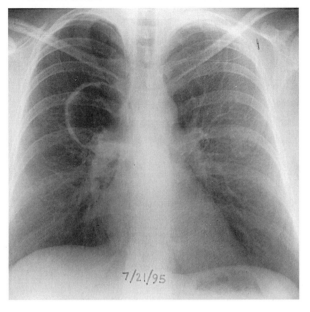

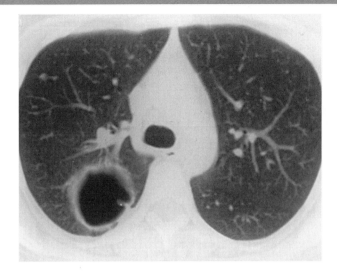

1. This patient reports recent travel to the southwestern United States. What is the most likely infectious etiology of this cavity?

2. Where else is this organism endemic?

3. Are cavities associated with the initial pneumonic form or the chronic form of this infection?

4. What is the typical pattern associated with disseminated coccidioidomycosis infection?

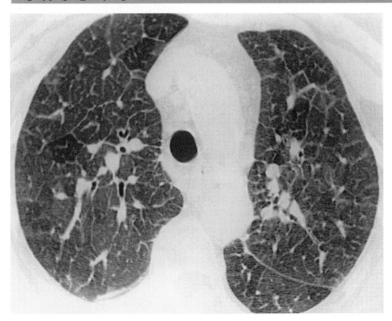

1. This patient's pulmonary venous wedge pressure was elevated. What is the most likely cause for these chest HRCT findings?

2. What chest radiographic finding correlates with the HRCT finding of thickened interlobular septa?

3. Define ground-glass opacity.

4. Name two technical features that are necessary components of HRCT imaging.

Cavity Due to Coccidioidomycosis

1. Coccidioidomycosis.

2. Central and South America and northern Mexico.

3. Chronic.

4. Multiple, small nodules.

Reference

Batra P, Batra RS: Thoracic coccidioidomycosis. *Semin Roentgenol* 31:28–44, 1996.

Cross-Reference

Thoracic Radiology: THE REQUISITES, p 125.

Comment

Coccidioidomycosis infection is caused by inhalation of infected spores of *Coccidioides immitis*, a soil inhabitant that is endemic to desert areas. Although most individuals are asymptomatic following exposure, some will experience a mild, flu-like illness.

Radiographic findings vary depending on the stage of infection. Following initial inhalation of the spores, there is a local pneumonic response, which is characterized radiographically as an area of consolidation. Such consolidation usually involves less than an entire lobe, is often located in the lower lobes, and usually resolves spontaneously without therapy.

Chronic pulmonary coccidioidomycosis is characterized radiographically by solitary or multiple pulmonary nodules and cavities. Such cavities, as demonstrated in this case, may have variable wall thickness and are usually radiologically indistinguishable from other causes of cavitary lesions. In a minority (10% to 15%) of cases, coccidioidomycosis is associated with characteristic thin-walled ("grapeskin") cavities. Such cavities may rapidly change in size, presumably due to a check-valve communication with the bronchial tree.

Disseminated coccidioidomycosis is rare; it presents radiographically as multiple nodules. The nodules usually range in size from 5 mm to 1 cm in diameter, but smaller miliary nodules may be observed in some cases. The course of disseminated coccidioidomycosis is variable: it may be chronic and insidious or rapidly fatal. The latter usually occurs in patients who are immunocompromised.

Notes

Hydrostatic Pulmonary Edema

1. Hydrostatic pulmonary edema.

2. Kerley (septal) lines.

3. Amorphous increase in lung attenuation that does not obscure pulmonary vessels.

4. Narrow collimation (1- to 2-mm) and high-resolution (bone) reconstruction algorithm.

Reference

Storto ML, Kee ST, Golden JA, Webb WR: Hydrostatic pulmonary edema: high-resolution CT findings. *AJR Am J Roentgenol* 165:817–820, 1995.

Cross-Reference

Thoracic Radiology: THE REQUISITES, pp 407–412.

Comment

Although a diagnosis of congestive heart failure is usually made on the basis of typical clinical and radiographic findings, occasionally patients with unsuspected congestive heart failure are imaged with chest HRCT in search of a cause of dyspnea. Hydrostatic edema is also an occasional incidental finding in patients who are being scanned for other purposes. Thus, it is important to be aware of the typical HRCT features of hydrostatic edema.

On HRCT of patients with hydrostatic edema, you may observe a combination of ground-glass opacity, smoothly thickened septal lines, peribronchovascular interstitial thickening, increased vascular caliber, and thickened fissures. Small pleural effusions, often right-sided, are also frequently observed. There is an absence of signs of fibrosis such as honeycombing, traction bronchiectasis, and architectural distortion. Interestingly, patients with acute congestive heart failure have also been reported to demonstrate occasionally enlarged mediastinal lymph nodes and haziness of the mediastinal fat.

Correlation between imaging findings and clinical data is usually sufficient to confirm the diagnosis. When the diagnosis is in doubt clinically, a follow-up study after diuresis can occasionally be helpful to confirm resolution of abnormalities and to exclude chronic infiltrative lung disease.

Notes

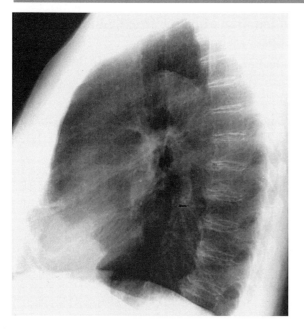
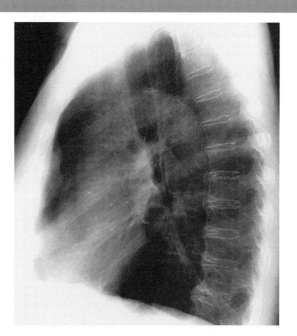

1. In this patient with a history of breast cancer, what is the most likely cause for the lobulated retrosternal opacity seen on the lateral chest radiograph in the second figure?

2. What other neoplastic process commonly involves this nodal group?

3. Does a normal chest radiograph exclude enlarged nodes at this site?

4. Name the most common site of enlarged nodes in patients with breast cancer.

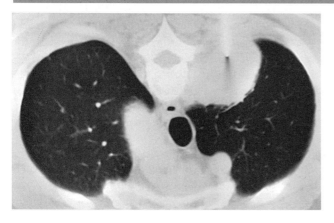
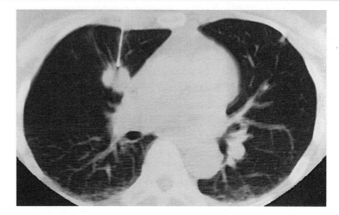

1. The figures are CT images of two different patients undergoing transthoracic needle biopsy (TTNB) procedures. Which patient is least likely to experience a pneumothorax from this procedure? Why?

2. What is the sensitivity of TTNB for malignant nodules?

3. Name at least three complications of TTNB.

4. How can you improve the yield of TTNB for diagnosing benign lesions?

Internal Mammary Lymph Node Enlargement

1. Enlarged internal mammary lymph nodes.

2. Lymphoma.

3. No.

4. Axilla.

Reference

Proto AV, Speckman JM: The left lateral radiograph of the chest. In: *Medical Radiography and Photography*, Vol 56. Rochester, NY, Eastman Kodak, 1980, 3:48–56.

Cross-Reference

Thoracic Radiology: THE REQUISITES, pp 467–478.

Comment

The serial lateral chest radiographs reveal interval development of a lobulated opacity in the retrosternal region. In a patient with a history of breast cancer, the most likely etiology is enlarged internal mammary lymph nodes, a common site of metastatic disease in such patients.

Enlarged internal mammary nodes are generally visible on chest radiographs only when they are considerably enlarged. On a posteroanterior (PA) chest radiograph of a patient with enlarged internal mammary nodes, you may observe a focal parasternal opacity, which is usually seen at the level of the first 3 intercostal spaces and less frequently at the fourth or fifth level. On a lateral radiograph, you may observe a lobulated retrosternal opacity, as demonstrated in this case. Most often, the opacity is observed at a more superior level than is shown in this case (e.g., see Fig. 17–11 in *Thoracic Radiology: THE REQUISITES*).

A lobulated retrosternal opacity may also be observed in patients with dilated internal mammary vessels. For example, coarctation of the aorta is associated with collateral internal mammary arteries and SVC obstruction is associated with collateral internal mammary veins. The former is associated with a characteristic appearance of the aorta and evidence of rib notching, and the latter is usually associated with a large mass in the right paratracheal region.

Notes

CT-guided Transthoracic Needle Biopsy Procedure

1. The patient in the first figure, because the needle does not traverse aerated lung.

2. Greater than 90%.

3. Pneumothorax (20% to 30%); chest tube (5% to 15%); hemoptysis (1% to 10%); seeding of biopsy track; and air embolism.

4. Use a cutting core biopsy needle that provides a histologic specimen.

Reference

Mason AC, Templeton PA: Transthoracic needle biopsy of the lung. *Appl Radiol* 7–12, 1996.

Cross-Reference

Thoracic Radiology: THE REQUISITES, pp 515–520.

Comment

The CT images demonstrate TTNB procedures of two separate patients. Note that the peripheral mass in the first figure does not require the biopsy needle to traverse aerated lung. Such lesions are associated with a very low pneumothorax rate.

With regard to planning a TTNB procedure, you should first obtain a prebiopsy CT scan. The shortest, most vertical route should be chosen, and the path of the needle should avoid interlobar fissures, pulmonary vessels, bullae, and areas of severe emphysema.

TTNB is a relatively safe and accurate procedure for obtaining biopsy specimens of lung nodules and masses. The sensitivity for malignant nodules is greater than 90%, and the accuracy for differentiating among various cell types of lung cancer is roughly 80%. A major limitation of TTNB using fine-needle aspiration is a relatively low sensitivity (10% to 40%) for making a specific benign diagnosis. However, this ability can be significantly improved by using core needle biopsy devices. Such devices provide histologic specimens that improve the accuracy of diagnosing benign entities such as granulomas, hamartomas, and organizing pneumonia.

It is important to remember that a negative biopsy for malignancy is not diagnostic unless a specific benign diagnosis has been rendered. Indeed, about 30% of nonspecific negative biopsies prove to represent malignancy. Thus, when you receive a nonspecific negative biopsy, you should consider repeating the biopsy with a core biopsy device.

Notes

Challenge

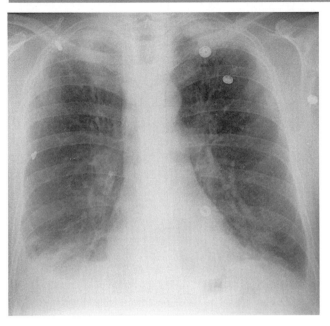 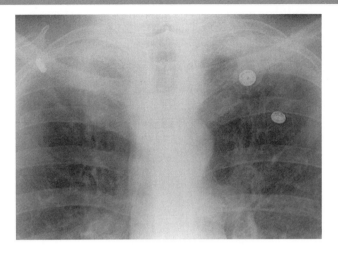

1. Name at least three entities that typically present with a peripheral distribution of consolidation.
2. Which entity is most closely associated with a "photographic negative of pulmonary edema" pattern?
3. How is this disorder treated?
4. What percentage of patients with chronic eosinophilic pneumonia have a history of asthma?

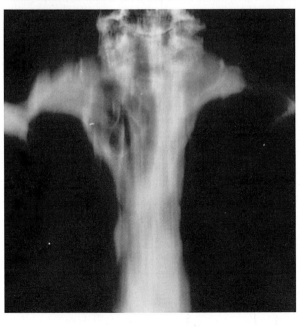 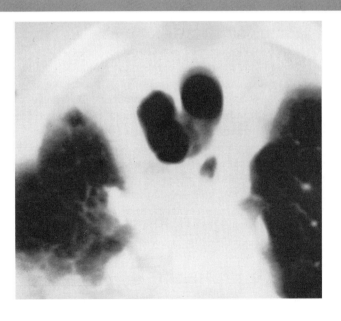

1. Name the structure that communicates with this cyst.
2. Is this a common location for this entity?
3. How can you differentiate this structure from an apical lung hernia?
4. What lung disorder is most closely associated with paratracheal air cysts?

Chronic Eosinophilic Pneumonia

1. Löffler's syndrome, chronic eosinophilic pneumonia, bronchiolitis obliterans organizing pneumonia (BOOP), pulmonary infarcts, vasculitides.

2. Chronic eosinophilic pneumonia.

3. Steroids.

4. About 50%.

Reference

Wilson AG: Immunologic diseases of the lungs. In: Armstrong P, Wilson AG, Dee P, Hansell DM, Eds: *Imaging of Diseases of the Chest*, second edition. St. Louis, Mosby, 1995, pp 526-527.

Cross-Reference

Thoracic Radiology: THE REQUISITES, pp 266-270.

Comment

The chest radiograph in this case demonstrates multifocal areas of consolidation in both lungs, with a striking peripheral predominance in the upper lobes (best demonstrated on the coned-down image in the second figure). The distribution is typical of chronic eosinophilic pneumonia.

Affected patients typically present with symptoms of dyspnea, fever, chills, night sweats, and weight loss. Women are affected more frequently than men, and there is a history of asthma in about one half of cases. Eosinophilia is present in the majority of patients.

The typical radiographic appearance is a peripheral pattern of consolidation, often with an apical or axillary distribution. The lung bases are less frequently involved. Also note the presence of right basilar consolidation in the first figure. In some patients, the opacities resolve and recur in the same location. When peripheral consolidation surrounds the lungs, the pattern is referred to as a photographic negative of pulmonary edema. Pleural effusions (which are present in this case) are infrequently encountered.

Affected patients usually show a rapid response to steroid therapy, with clinical improvement within hours and radiographic resolution within days.

Notes

Right Paratracheal Air Cyst (Diverticulum)

1. Trachea.

2. Yes.

3. Only an apical lung hernia is contiguous with the lung and demonstrates lung architectural features.

4. Emphysema.

Reference

Goo JM, Im J, Ahn JM, et al: Right paratracheal air cysts in the thoracic inlet: clinical and radiologic significance. *AJR Am J Roentgenol* 173:65-70, 1999.

Cross-Reference

None.

Comment

The conventional tomogram in the first figure demonstrates a well-marginated, septated cystic structure in the right paratracheal region adjacent to the right lung apex. The differential diagnosis includes a right paratracheal air cyst, apical bullae, and an apical lung hernia. The CT image in the second figure demonstrates that the cystic structure is mediastinal in location, directly communicates with the right posterolateral wall of the trachea, and does not demonstrate lung architectural features. The imaging characteristics are typical of a right paratracheal air cyst, a rare abnormality of the trachea that is thought to represent a tracheal diverticulum.

Such diverticula occur most commonly at the right posterolateral wall of the trachea at the level of the thoracic inlet. Interestingly, tracheal diverticula have been reported to have an association with chronic respiratory disorders, most notably emphysema. It has been proposed that tracheal diverticula occur in response to raised intratracheal pressures related to repeated bouts of coughing. Presenting clinical symptoms of tracheal diverticula include prolonged productive cough, hemoptysis, and chest pain. Symptomatic lesions are treated surgically.

Notes

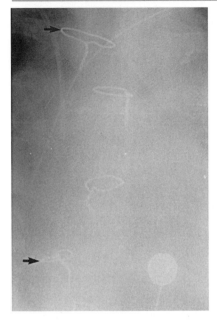

1. What postoperative complication is present in this case?
2. Is this a serious complication?
3. How is this complication treated?
4. What sternal wire abnormality is most commonly seen on postoperative radiographs in patients with this complication?

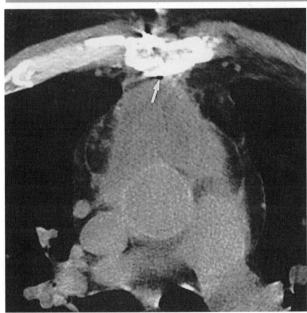

1. What is the most likely cause for the mediastinal fluid collection in this septic patient who is 18 days status post median sternotomy?
2. In the postoperative setting, are the CT findings of localized retrosternal fluid collections and pneumomediastinum highly sensitive for mediastinitis?
3. Are these findings highly specific in the early postoperative period?
4. At what time point after surgery does the specificity of this finding increase?

Sternal Dehiscence Following Median Sternotomy

1. Sternal dehiscence.

2. Yes.

3. Reoperation for sternal closure.

4. Sternal wire displacement.

Reference

Boiselle PM, Mansilla AV, Fisher MS, McLoud TC: Wandering wires: frequency of sternal wire abnormalities in patients with sternal dehiscence. *AJR Am J Roentgenol* 173:777-780, 1999.

Cross-Reference

None.

Comment

Following median sternotomy, the sternal wires are typically maintained in a vertical row along the midline of the sternum. The coned-down chest radiograph shows a scrambled arrangement of the sternal wires, with the first and fourth wires displaced to the right of the midline *(arrows)*. Displacement of sternal wires is a highly sensitive and specific sign for sternal dehiscence, an uncommon but serious complication following median sternotomy.

Although sternal dehiscence is often evident on the basis of physical examination findings, it may be clinically occult in some cases. Sternal wire abnormalities, most notably displacement, are seen in the majority of patients with this condition; importantly, such abnormalities may precede the clinical diagnosis in some cases. Thus, when reviewing postoperative radiographs of a patient who is status post median sternotomy, you should carefully assess the sternal wires. Interval displacement or rotation of one or more wires (in comparison with their appearance on the first postoperative radiograph) should prompt careful clinical assessment for signs of dehiscence.

The high frequency of sternal wire displacement in patients with sternal dehiscence fits well with the proposed mechanism of this complication. It has been proposed that sternal separation is the result of sternal sutures pulling or cutting through the sternum rather than breaking. As the sternum separates, some sutures will travel with the right side of the sternum and others will migrate to the left side. The term *wandering wires* has been used to describe the characteristic alterations in sternal wires on radiographs of patients with sternal dehiscence.

Notes

Postoperative Mediastinitis

1. Mediastinitis.

2. Yes.

3. No.

4. After 14 days.

Reference

Jolles H, Henry DA, Robertson JF, Cole TJ, Spratt JA: Mediastinitis following median sternotomy: CT findings. *Radiology* 201:463-466, 1996.

Cross-Reference

Thoracic Radiology: THE REQUISITES, pp 464-466.

Comment

Mediastinitis is a relatively uncommon but serious complication following median sternotomy. Mediastinitis refers to inflammation and infection of the mediastinum and is a more serious complication than superficial infection localized to the peristernal soft tissue structures of the chest wall.

The CT diagnosis of mediastinitis is based primarily on the presence of mediastinal air and fluid collections. It is important to be aware that such findings can be seen normally in the early postoperative period in patients without mediastinitis.

In a study of patients with postoperative mediastinitis by Jolles and colleagues, it was reported that the CT findings of localized mediastinal fluid and pneumomediastinum *(arrow)* are highly sensitive (100%) for mediastinitis. The specificity of these findings is quite low (33%) within the first 14 days following surgery but increases significantly (100%) after postoperative day 14. Thus, when evaluating the CT scan of a postoperative patient with suspected mediastinitis, you must correlate CT findings with the time interval since surgery.

Although these data suggest that CT is most helpful in the late postoperative period, there is a role for CT imaging in the early postoperative period as well. For example, a negative CT scan of the mediastinum can be useful for directing attention to other sites of possible infection. Moreover, the identification of localized retrosternal fluid collections may be helpful for guiding aspiration procedures in patients in whom there is a strong clinical suspicion for mediastinitis.

Notes

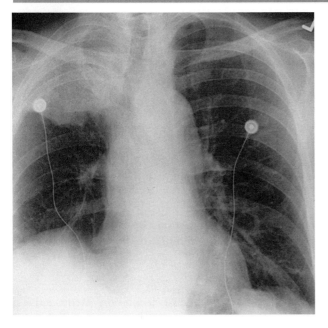
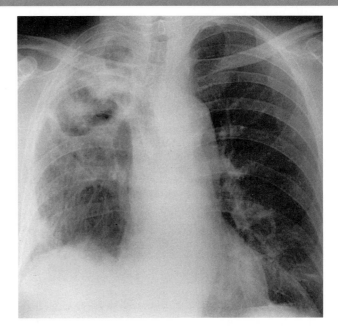

1. What is the most likely cause for these serial radiographic findings that developed within 1 week following right upper lobe resection for lung cancer?

2. What type of organism is most commonly responsible for nosocomial pneumonia?

3. What term is used to describe cavitary pneumonia associated with intracavitary sloughed lung?

4. What organism is most closely associated with this entity?

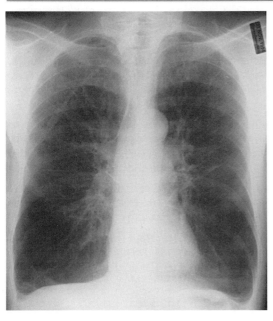
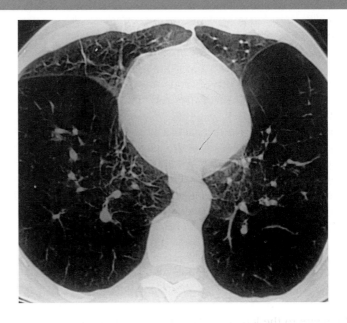

1. What is the distribution of emphysema in this patient?

2. Is this distribution typical of emphysema related to cigarette smoking?

3. Name the four basic types of emphysema.

4. Name at least one cause of panlobular emphysema with a basilar predominance.

C A S E 1 0 2

Pulmonary Gangrene Secondary to *Klebsiella* Pneumonia

1. Pneumonia.

2. Gram-negative organisms.

3. Pulmonary gangrene.

4. *Klebsiella.*

Reference

Armstrong P, Dee P: Infections in the lung and pleura. In: Armstrong P, Wilson AG, Dee P, Hansell DM, Eds: *Imaging of Diseases of the Chest*, second edition. St. Louis, Mosby, 1995, p 149.

Cross-Reference

Thoracic Radiology: THE REQUISITES, pp 103–104.

Comment

Nosocomial pneumonia is most commonly caused by gram-negative organisms. Hospitalized patients at increased risk for nosocomial pneumonia include patients who are maintained on artificial ventilators and those who have intravenous catheters and other forms of ancillary support devices.

Pneumonia may be complicated by lung necrosis and cavitation, particularly when it is caused by virulent organisms. Bacteria that frequently cause cavitation include *Staphylococcus aureus*, gram-negative bacteria, anaerobic bacteria, and *Mycobacterium tuberculosis*. When necrosis is extensive, arteritis and vascular thrombosis may develop in an area of intense inflammation, resulting in ischemic necrosis and death of a portion of the lung. This process may result in the presence of sloughed lung within a cavity (second figure) and is referred to as pulmonary gangrene. You should not confuse this entity with the "ball-in-cavity" appearance that is associated with the saprophytic form of *Aspergillus* infection. An aspergilloma develops within a long-standing, preexisting cavity. In contrast, in pulmonary gangrene, a cavity and intracavitary sloughed lung develop rapidly within an area of acute consolidation.

Although pulmonary gangrene is most closely associated with *Klebsiella*, it is not specific for this organism. This entity has been described in association with a variety of other organisms, including *Streptococcus pneumoniae*, *M. tuberculosis*, and *Mucormycetes*.

Notes

C A S E 1 0 3

Panlobular Emphysema Secondary to Intravenous Methylphenidate

1. Lower lobe predominance.

2. No.

3. Centrilobular, panlobular, paraseptal, and paracicatricial.

4. Alpha$_1$-antitrypsin (AAT) deficiency and intravenous injection of methylphenidate (Ritalin).

Reference

Stern EJ, Frank MS, Schmutz JF, et al: Panlobular pulmonary emphysema caused by IV injection of methylphenidate (Ritalin): findings on chest radiographs and CT scans. *AJR Am J Roentgenol* 162:555–560, 1994.

Cross-Reference

Thoracic Radiology: THE REQUISITES, pp 287–295.

Comment

Emphysema is defined by the presence of abnormal, permanent enlargement of the airspaces distal to the terminal bronchiole, accompanied by destruction of their walls without obvious fibrosis.

The radiograph demonstrates hyperinflation of the lungs with associated reduced vascularity in the lower lobes. The high-resolution CT (HRCT) image reveals extensive areas of abnormal low attenuation in the lower lobes with a paucity of pulmonary vessels. The CT appearance is typical of panlobular emphysema, which has been described as a "diffuse simplification of lung architecture." Panlobular emphysema is almost always most severe in the lower lobes. In contrast, centrilobular emphysema is usually most prominent in the upper lobes.

AAT deficiency is the most common cause of panlobular emphysema with a lower lobe predominance. Intravenous drug abusers who inject methylphenidate may develop a basilar distribution of panlobular emphysema that is indistinguishable radiographically from AAT deficiency. The pathogenesis of emphysema in such patients is unknown. This condition can be distinguished from AAT deficiency by a history of methylphenidate injection, normal AAT serum levels, and pathologic evidence of microscopic talc granulomas.

Notes

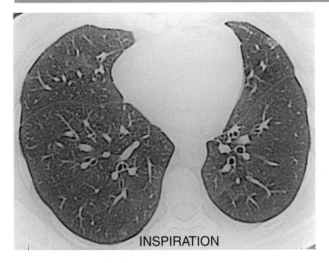

INSPIRATION

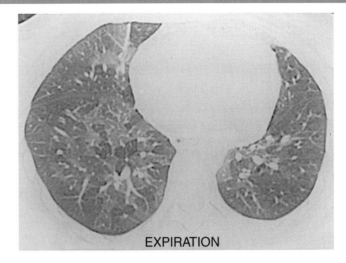

EXPIRATION

1. In a patient who is status post bone marrow transplantation, what is the most likely cause for these inspiratory and expiratory HRCT findings?

2. Name three CT findings that may be associated with bronchiolitis obliterans (BO).

3. Is BO a constrictive or a proliferative form of bronchiolitis?

4. Name at least four diseases or conditions that may be associated with BO.

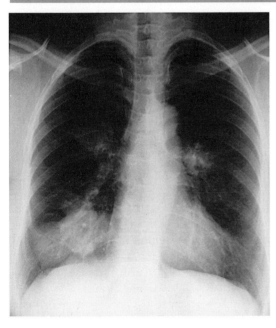

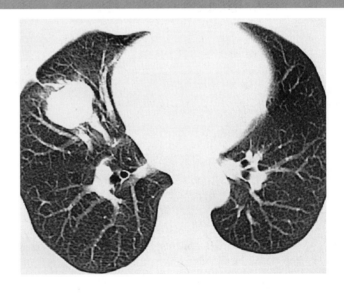

1. Name the condition that is characterized by multiple pulmonary nodules and masses in a patient who is status post prior hysterectomy for uterine fibroids.

2. What is the typical growth pattern for pulmonary lesions associated with this condition?

3. Name another neoplasm that is characterized by extremely slowly growing pulmonary metastases.

4. Name at least two neoplasms that are associated with rapidly growing pulmonary metastases.

CASE 104

Bronchiolitis Obliterans

1. BO.

2. Mosaic perfusion, bronchial dilation, and air trapping.

3. Constrictive.

4. Bone marrow transplantation, viral infections, toxic fume inhalation, rheumatoid arthritis, lung transplantation, and inflammatory bowel disease.

Reference

Worthy SA, Flint JD, Müller NL: Pulmonary complications after bone marrow transplantation: high-resolution CT and pathologic findings. *Radiographics* 17:1359–1371, 1997.

Cross-Reference

Thoracic Radiology: THE REQUISITES, pp 396–400.

Comment

The inspiratory HRCT image in the first figure reveals a subtle pattern of variable lung attenuation, with a slight decrease in the caliber and number of pulmonary vessels within the areas of low attenuation. This appearance has been referred to as a "mosaic pattern" of lung attenuation and may be encountered in patients with small airways disease and pulmonary vascular abnormalities such as chronic pulmonary embolism. The expiratory HRCT image in the second figure demonstrates extensive air trapping, a finding that distinguishes small airways disease from pulmonary vascular disease.

A mosaic pattern of lung attenuation with air trapping on expiratory scans is the hallmark of BO. BO is characterized histologically by concentric narrowing of the bronchioles by submucosal and peribronchiolar fibrosis. Affected patients typically present with dyspnea. Pulmonary function tests reveal a progressive, nonreversible airflow obstruction pattern.

A variety of conditions are associated with BO, including bone marrow transplantation. Approximately 10% of bone marrow transplant patients develop BO. In such patients, BO is thought to be related to chronic graft-versus-host disease and has a high mortality rate.

Notes

CASE 105

Metastasizing Leiomyoma

1. Metastasizing leiomyoma.

2. Slowly growing.

3. Thyroid carcinoma.

4. Sarcomas, melanomas, and germ cell neoplasms.

Reference

Armstrong P: Neoplasms of the lungs, airways, and pleura. In: Armstrong P, Wilson AG, Dee P, Hansell DM, Eds: *Imaging of Diseases of the Chest*, second edition. St. Louis, Mosby, 1995, p 317.

Cross-Reference

Thoracic Radiology: THE REQUISITES, pp 334–340.

Comment

Pulmonary metastases are an important cause of multiple lung nodules and masses. Such nodules and masses are usually peripheral in location and have a basilar predominance.

Leiomyomas are an uncommon cause of pulmonary metastases. The behavior of such lesions varies from that of a benign lesion to a low-grade sarcoma. Thus, the more general term *metastasizing leiomyoma* is preferable to the phrase *benign metastasizing leiomyoma*.

In women, these lesions may be very slowly growing metastases from a uterine leiomyoma. Affected patients often have a history of previous hysterectomy for uterine fibroids. The pulmonary lesions are usually very sensitive to hormonal therapy.

Notes

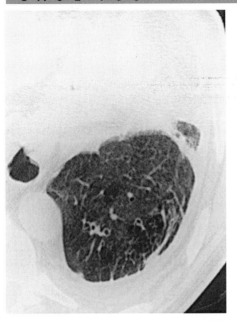
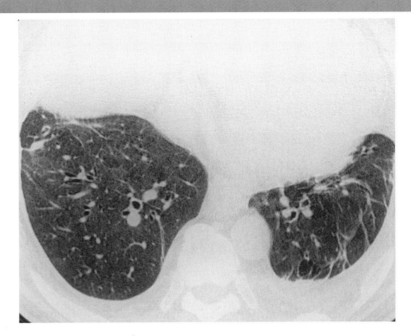

1. What is the term used to describe the curvilinear opacity in the first figure that courses parallel to the pleural surface?
2. What is the term used to describe the long linear opacities in the second figure that course perpendicular to the pleural surface?
3. With what chronic infiltrative lung disease are these findings most closely associated?
4. Are they pathognomonic for this process?

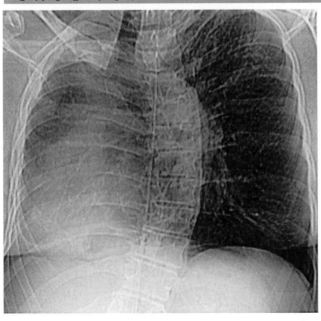
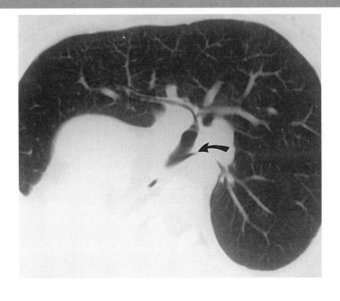

1. In this patient with a history of prior right pneumonectomy, how can you explain the presence of aerated lung in the right hemithorax?
2. Why do you think that this patient is experiencing dyspnea?
3. Is the postpneumonectomy syndrome more common following right or left pneumonectomy?
4. How is this syndrome treated?

Asbestosis

1. Subpleural line.

2. Parenchymal bands.

3. Asbestosis.

4. No.

Reference

Staples CA: Computed tomography in the evaluation of benign asbestos-related disorders. *Radiol Clin North Am* 30:1191–1207, 1992.

Cross-Reference

Thoracic Radiology: THE REQUISITES, pp 238–241.

Comment

Asbestosis refers to pulmonary fibrosis that occurs in asbestos workers. It usually occurs in individuals who have been exposed to high concentrations over a prolonged period. Affected patients typically present with symptoms of a dry cough and dyspnea. Pulmonary function tests reveal a progressive reduction in vital capacity and diffusing capacity.

On conventional radiographs, you may observe a linear or reticular pattern of parenchymal opacities in the lower lung zones, which may progress to honeycombing. The identification of pleural plaques or pleural thickening supports the diagnosis (note pleural thickening in the figures). However, pleural abnormalities may be absent. It is important to recognize that normal conventional radiographs do not exclude a diagnosis of asbestosis.

CT, particularly HRCT, is superior to radiography in the detection, quantification, and characterization of asbestosis. HRCT findings include (1) curvilinear subpleural lines; (2) thickened septal lines (the most common finding); (3) subpleural dependent density; (4) parenchymal bands; and (5) honeycombing. In an asbestos-exposed individual with a normal chest radiograph, these HRCT findings are suggestive of asbestosis; however, they are not specific for this process.

Notes

Postpneumonectomy Syndrome

1. Herniation of the left upper lobe into the right hemithorax.

2. Compression of the left lower lobe bronchus by vascular structures.

3. Right.

4. Surgical repositioning of the mediastinal structures.

Reference

Boiselle PM, Shepard JO, McLoud TC, Grillo HC, Wright CD: Postpneumonectomy syndrome: another twist. *J Thorac Imaging* 12:209–211, 1997.

Cross-Reference

None.

Comment

Postpneumonectomy syndrome is a rare, delayed complication following pneumonectomy, often performed at an early age. It is more common following right pneumonectomy than left pneumonectomy. Affected patients present with symptoms of dyspnea and recurrent infections in the remaining lung.

The syndrome occurs secondary to marked mediastinal shift, rotation of the heart and great vessels, and herniation of the remaining lung into the contralateral side of the chest. Following realignment of these structures, the airway may be compressed (*arrow*, second figure) by the thoracic spine, descending thoracic aorta, ligamentum arteriosum, and pulmonary artery.

CT plays an important role in delineating the presence and cause of airway obstruction. Inspiratory-expiratory CT may also assess for the presence of tracheobronchomalacia, an important preoperative finding. Prompt diagnosis and treatment are important, because surgical results are favorable before malacic changes have occurred within the obstructed airway.

Notes

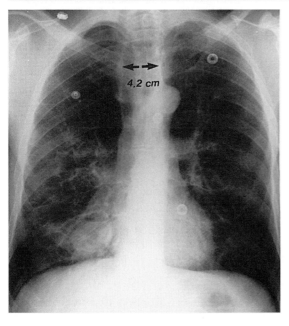

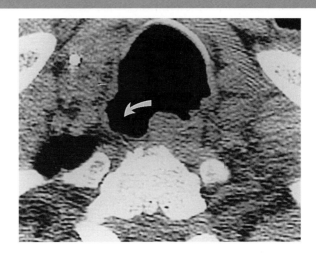

1. What is Mounier-Kuhn syndrome?
2. What is the radiologic definition of tracheomegaly?
3. What does the curved arrow in the second figure represent?
4. Is this a common location for this finding?

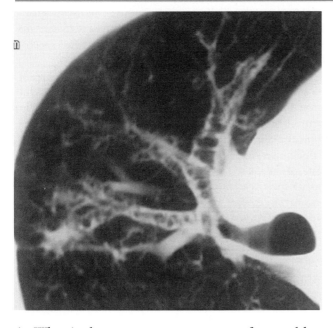

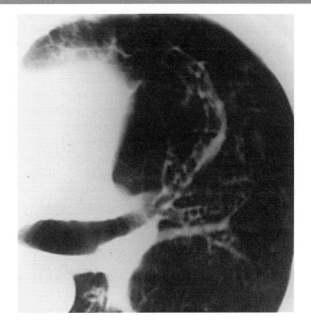

1. What is the most common cause of central bronchiectasis?
2. What other imaging findings are associated with allergic bronchopulmonary aspergillosis (ABPA)?
3. What types of patients are predisposed to this condition?
4. Characterize the type of bronchiectasis in this case (cylindrical, varicose, or cystic).

Mounier-Kuhn Syndrome With Tracheal Diverticulum

1. An entity characterized by congenital tracheobronchomegaly and recurrent respiratory infections.

2. A coronal tracheal diameter of greater than 25 mm, as measured 2 cm above the aortic arch on a standard posteroanterior (PA) erect chest radiograph

3. A tracheal diverticulum.

4. Yes.

Reference
Woodring JH, Howard RS, Rehm SR: Congenital tracheo-bronchomegaly (Mounier-Kuhn syndrome): a report of 10 cases and review of the literature. *J Thorac Imaging* 6:1–10, 1991.

Cross-Reference
Thoracic Radiology: THE REQUISITES, pp 68–69, 362, 364.

Comment
Mounier-Kuhn syndrome, also referred to as congenital tracheobronchomegaly, is characterized pathologically by atrophy or absence of elastic fibers and thinning of the muscular mucosa of the trachea and main bronchi. This results in a flaccid airway that abnormally dilates during inspiration and excessively collapses on expiration. An ineffective coughing mechanism and pooling of secretions within outpouchings of mucosa predispose affected patients to recurrent bouts of respiratory infections. Pulmonary complications include bronchiectasis, emphysema, and pulmonary fibrosis. Note the presence of tracheomegaly (note 4.2 cm diameter coronal dimension), cystic bronchiectasis, and emphysema in the first figure.

The second figure reveals an enlarged trachea and a wide-mouthed tracheal diverticulum *(curved arrow)*. The posterolateral wall of the trachea is the most common location for a diverticulum in patients with Mounier-Kuhn syndrome. This site represents the junction of the posterior membranous and the anterior cartilaginous portions of the trachea.

Notes

Allergic Bronchopulmonary Aspergillosis

1. Allergic bronchopulmonary aspergillosis (ABPA).

2. Mucoid impaction, recurrent atelectasis, patchy consolidation.

3. Asthmatics.

4. Varicose.

Reference
Miller WT: Aspergillosis: a disease with many faces. *Semin Roentgenol* 31:52–66, 1996.

Cross-Reference
Thoracic Radiology: THE REQUISITES, pp 129, 298, 394, 396.

Comment
ABPA is a hypersensitivity reaction that occurs when *Aspergillus* organisms are inhaled by an atopic individual. The inhaled fungus grows in a noninvasive manner within the bronchi and incites an allergic response. The bronchi become dilated and filled with mucus that contains abundant eosinophils and fragmented fungal hyphae.

Affected patients typically have a history of asthma. Presenting signs and symptoms may include fever, pleuritic chest pain, expectoration of mucous plugs, and chronic cough. Radiographic features include central bronchiectasis; mucous plugging ("finger-in-glove" appearance); atelectasis; and patchy, migratory foci of consolidation.

The most characteristic finding is mucous plugging. As the mucous plugs are expectorated, dilated, air-filled bronchi can be identified, especially on CT scans. The central bronchi are most commonly affected, and they typically demonstrate a varicoid appearance.

Because ABPA is an allergic disease, treatment consists of steroids. Chronic cases may be complicated by upper lobe scarring and bronchiectasis.

Notes

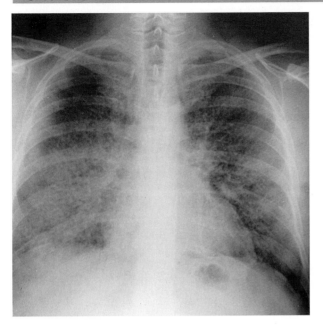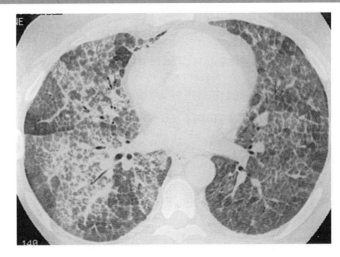

1. What HRCT findings are associated with the term *crazy paving*?
2. Name the disorder that is classically associated with this pattern.
3. Name three types of pulmonary infections that may complicate pulmonary alveolar proteinosis (PAP).
4. How is PAP treated?

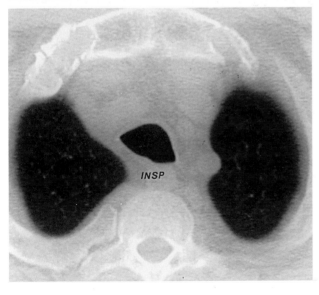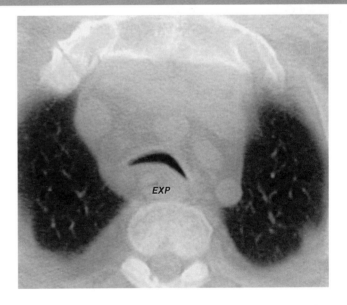

1. Define tracheomalacia.
2. What do patients with primary (congenital) tracheomalacia lack?
3. During which phase of respiration is tracheal collapsibility most apparent?
4. What percentage of tracheal luminal narrowing during respiration is considered abnormal?

Pulmonary Alveolar Proteinosis

1. Ground-glass opacity with superimposed smooth septal thickening in a patchy or geographic distribution.

2. Pulmonary alveolar proteinosis (PAP).

3. Infection with *Nocardia*, *Aspergillus*, and *Mucormycetes*.

4. Bronchoalveolar lavage.

Reference
Webb WR, Müller NL, Naidich DP: *High-Resolution CT of the Lung*, second edition. Philadelphia, Lippincott-Raven, 1996, pp 202-203.

Cross-Reference
Thoracic Radiology: THE REQUISITES, pp 223-225.

Comment
PAP is characterized by filling of the alveolar spaces with periodic acid–Schiff (PAS)-positive proteinaceous material, with little or no associated tissue reaction. Although most cases are idiopathic, PAP has been reported to occur in association with an overwhelming exposure to silica and in association with immunologic disturbances.

PAP typically affects men in the fourth and fifth decades of life, and presenting symptoms include a nonproductive cough and dyspnea. Chest radiographic findings are often striking and consist of alveolar consolidation and ground-glass opacification in a symmetric, bilateral, perihilar distribution. On HRCT, ground-glass opacification predominates, and it is often patchy or geographic. A "crazy paving" pattern is formed when smoothly thickened septal lines are superimposed on ground-glass opacification.

The prognosis of PAP has improved since the advent of therapy with bronchoalveolar lavage, which is successful in most cases. However, some patients require retreatment for relapse, and a minority of patients eventually become refractory to treatment.

Notes

Tracheomalacia

1. Excessive collapsibility of the trachea secondary to weakness of the tracheal walls and supporting cartilages.

2. Cartilage.

3. Expiration.

4. Greater than 50% of narrowing.

Reference
Suto Y, Tanabe Y: Evaluation of tracheal collapsibility in patients with tracheomalacia using dynamic MR imaging during coughing. *AJR Am J Roentgenol* 171:393-394, 1998.

Cross-Reference
Thoracic Radiology: THE REQUISITES, pp 369-370.

Comment
Tracheobronchomalacia refers to excessive collapsibility of the airway. Such collapsibility is usually most apparent during coughing and at forced expiration. The abnormally flaccid airway is associated with physiologic alterations, including an inefficient coughing mechanism and retained secretions. This may lead to recurrent infections and bronchiectasis.

A primary cause of tracheobronchomalacia is congenital deficiency of cartilage. Acquired causes include intubation, chronic obstructive pulmonary disease, trauma, infection, relapsing polychondritis, and extrinsic compression (e.g., from a thyroid goiter).

The diagnosis is made by comparing the airway lumen diameter at inspiration (INSP) with the diameter at either forced expiration (EXP) or during coughing. This can be performed by a variety of imaging methods, including fluoroscopy, cine CT, inspiration/expiration CT, and dynamic MRI. Normally, the airway lumen shows a decrease of approximately 10% to 30% with expiration or coughing. A decrease of greater than 50% is generally considered abnormal.

Notes

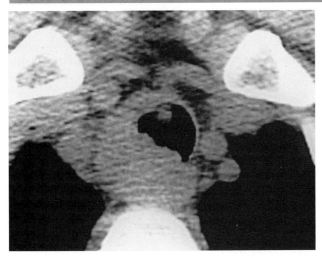
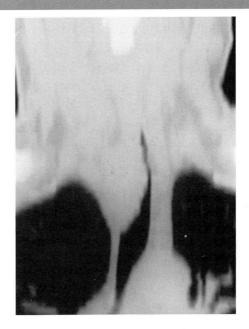

1. What are the two most common cell types of primary malignant tracheal neoplasms?

2. Which of the two cell types is more common in cigarette smokers?

3. Which of the two cell types has a better prognosis?

4. In general, what degree of tracheal luminal narrowing must be present before patients are symptomatic from a primary tracheal malignancy?

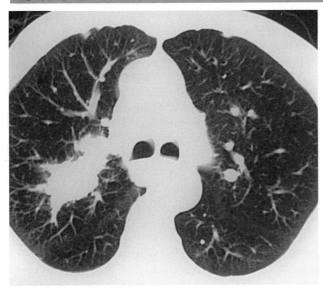
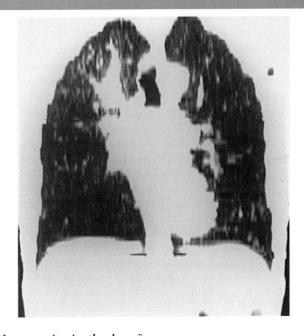

1. What are the two most common causes of a tubular opacity in the lung?

2. List two entities that are commonly associated with mucoid impaction.

3. What is the most common cell type of non-small cell lung cancer to present as an endobronchial lesion?

4. When mucoid impaction occurs secondary to bronchial obstruction, how does the adjacent lung remain aerated?

Adenoid Cystic Carcinoma of the Trachea

1. Squamous cell carcinoma and adenoid cystic carcinoma.

2. Squamous cell carcinoma.

3. Adenoid cystic carcinoma.

4. A reduction to approximately one third of the normal tracheal width.

Reference

McCarthy MJ, Rosado-de-Christenson ML: Tumors of the trachea. *J Thorac Imaging* 10:180–198, 1995.

Cross-Reference

Thoracic Radiology: THE REQUISITES, pp 364–369.

Comment

Primary tracheal neoplasms are quite rare. In adult patients, the majority of tracheal neoplasms are malignant. Presenting symptoms include shortness of breath and wheezing. Affected patients may be initially misdiagnosed with adult-onset asthma. This diagnosis should prompt you to carefully assess the airway on chest radiographs!

Squamous cell carcinoma has a male predilection, and it is strongly associated with cigarette smoking. Squamous cell carcinoma is associated with a poor prognosis. Therapy consists of surgery and radiation for localized disease and radiation alone for surgically unresectable cases.

Adenoid cystic carcinoma is a low-grade malignancy that has no gender predilection and no relationship to cigarette smoking. Adenoid cystic carcinoma has a significantly better prognosis than squamous cell carcinoma, and surgical resection is potentially curative for patients with localized disease. Late recurrences and metastases have been reported, however, especially among patients treated only with radiation therapy.

Notes

Mucoid Impaction Secondary to Bronchial Obstruction (Squamous Cell Carcinoma)

1. Mucoid impaction and arteriovenous malformation.

2. ABPA and cystic fibrosis.

3. Squamous cell carcinoma.

4. Collateral air drift.

Reference

Armstrong P: Basic patterns in lung disease. In: Armstrong P, Wilson AG, Dee P, Hansell DM, Eds: *Imaging of Diseases of the Chest*, second edition. St. Louis, Mosby, 1995, p 109.

Cross-Reference

Thoracic Radiology: THE REQUISITES, p 391.

Comment

Mucoid impaction results in the presence of branching, tubular Y- and V-shaped opacities, which are also referred to as a "finger-in-glove" appearance. Mucoid impaction is most often associated with ABPA and cystic fibrosis. It is important to be aware that mucoid impaction can also occur distal to a bronchial obstruction from both malignant (e.g., bronchogenic carcinoma, bronchial carcinoid) and benign (e.g., tuberculosis [TB] bronchostenosis) etiologies. In such cases, the affected portion of the lung remains aerated secondary to collateral air drift.

When you identify tubular opacities on a chest radiograph, you should consider both mucoid impaction and arteriovenous malformation as potential diagnoses. They can usually be distinguished on CT scans by assessing the bronchi. Only in cases of arteriovenous malformation is a normal bronchus observed adjacent to the tubular opacity. In some cases, low CT density numbers (-5 to $+20$) can confirm the diagnosis of mucoid impaction. If the diagnosis remains in doubt, contrast-enhanced CT can readily differentiate between these entities, because only an arteriovenous malformation enhances with contrast.

Notes

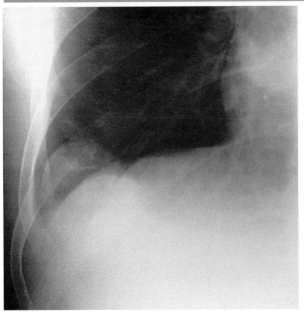
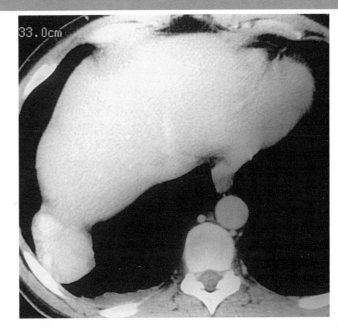

1. Are all localized fibrous tumors of the pleura histologically benign?
2. Are localized fibrous tumors of the pleura related to asbestos exposure?
3. Name a skeletal abnormality that is associated with fibrous tumors of the pleura.
4. What is the typical signal intensity of fibrous tumors of the pleura on T1W and T2W MRI?

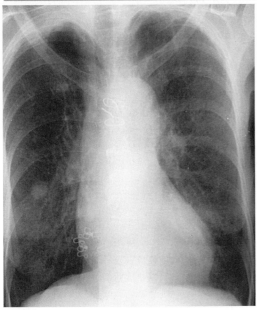
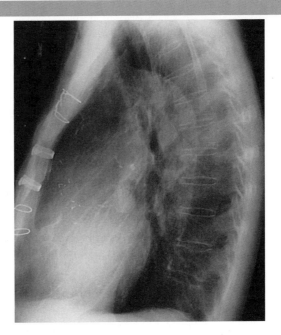

1. In a patient who is status post heart transplantation, is a pulmonary nodule or mass more likely to be neoplastic or infectious in etiology?
2. Infections with which two organisms comprise the majority of lung nodules or masses in heart transplant patients?
3. Name the most common noninfectious etiology of lung nodules or masses in heart transplant patients.
4. Approximately what percentage of heart transplant patients develop posttransplant lymphoproliferative disorder?

Localized Fibrous Tumor of the Pleura

1. No.

2. No.

3. Hypertrophic osteoarthropathy.

4. Low signal intensity on T1W and T2W.

Reference

Ferretti GR, Chiles C, Choplin RH, Coulomb M: Localized benign fibrous tumors of the pleura. *AJR Am J Roentgenol* 169:683–686, 1997.

Cross-Reference

Thoracic Radiology: THE REQUISITES, pp 502, 503.

Comment

Localized fibrous tumors of the pleura are uncommon primary pleural neoplasms. Histologically, approximately 60% are benign and 40% are malignant. However, all lesions are associated with a good prognosis, and the majority are curable by surgical resection.

Affected patients typically present in the sixth to seventh decades of life. In approximately 50% of cases, the patients are asymptomatic. Large lesions may produce symptoms such as cough, dyspnea, and chest pain. In a small minority of cases, patients may present with extrapulmonary manifestations, including hypertrophic osteoarthropathy and episodic hypoglycemia.

On chest radiographs, localized fibrous tumors of the pleura typically appear as round or lobulated masses. Such masses vary in size, and they typically demonstrate a slow growth rate. Lesions that are attached to the visceral pleura by a pedicle demonstrate mobility in response to changes in respiration and alterations in patient positioning.

On contrast-enhanced CT scans, fibrous lesions of the pleura typically demonstrate intense and homogeneous contrast enhancement (as shown in the second figure), reflecting the rich vascularization of these tumors. On MRI, these lesions typically demonstrate low signal intensity on all sequences, reflecting the fibrous content within the stroma of the tumor.

Notes

Solitary Pulmonary Nodule Secondary to *Nocardia* Infection in a Heart Transplant Patient

1. Infectious.

2. *Aspergillus* and *Nocardia*.

3. Posttransplant lymphoproliferative disorder.

4. 5%.

Reference

Haramati LB, Schulman LL, Austin JHM: Lung nodules and masses after cardiac transplantation. *Radiology* 188:491–497, 1993.

Cross-Reference

Thoracic Radiology: THE REQUISITES, pp 135–142.

Comment

Cardiac transplantation is currently a widely accepted treatment for end-stage heart disease. The most common causes of morbidity and mortality following heart transplantation are infection and rejection.

When you detect single or multiple lung nodules or masses in a patient who is status post heart transplantation, you should first consider infectious etiologies such as *Aspergillus* and *Nocardia*. In a series of 257 patients who underwent heart transplantation, single or multiple lung nodules or masses were detected on chest radiographs in approximately 10% of patients. Infections were the most common etiology, with *Aspergillus* encountered slightly more frequently than *Nocardia*. *Aspergillus* infection developed a median of 2 months following transplantation, whereas *Nocardia* infection developed a median of 5 months after transplantation.

Posttransplant lymphoproliferative disorder is an important noninfectious cause of lung nodules and masses. This disorder usually occurs at least 4 to 6 months following transplantation. Lung parenchymal abnormalities are frequently accompanied by mediastinal and/or hilar lymph node enlargement, a finding that is not typically associated with *Aspergillus* and *Nocardia* infections.

Notes

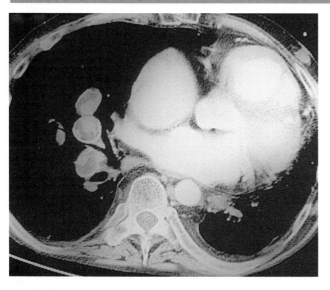
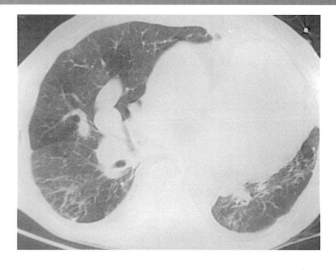

1. What is the most likely cause of pulmonary artery hypertension in this patient?

2. Name the term that is used to describe areas of variable lung attenuation with a lobular or multilobular distribution, as shown in the second figure?

3. Is mural thrombus a characteristic feature of acute or chronic pulmonary thromboembolism?

4. Is calcified thrombus a characteristic feature of acute or chronic pulmonary thromboembolism?

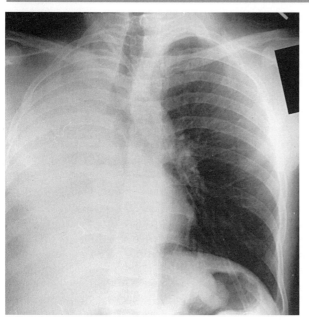
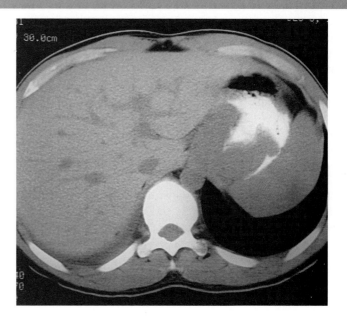

1. What is the reason for complete opacification of the right hemithorax in this young adult man?

2. Name at least four neoplastic causes of an endobronchial lesion.

3. What abnormality is present in the left upper quadrant in the second figure?

4. Name at least one malignant process that can result in an endobronchial lesion and gastric wall thickening.

C A S E   1 1 6

Chronic Pulmonary Thromboembolism

1. Chronic pulmonary thromboembolism.

2. Mosaic pattern.

3. Chronic.

4. Chronic.

Reference

Bergin CJ: Chronic thromboembolic pulmonary hypertension: the disease, the diagnosis, and the treatment. *Semin Ultrasound CT MRI* 18:383–391, 1997.

Cross-Reference

Thoracic Radiology: THE REQUISITES, pp 417–419.

Comment

Chronic pulmonary thromboembolism is a relatively uncommon but highly treatable cause of pulmonary artery hypertension. Because many affected patients do not present with a history of prior embolic episodes, the diagnosis may be difficult to make clinically.

Helical CT is playing an increasingly prominent role in the diagnosis of chronic pulmonary thromboembolism. Characteristic findings have been described in the lung parenchyma and pulmonary vessels. With regard to the lung parenchyma, you may observe variable areas of lung attenuation, with a lobular or multilobular distribution, referred to as a mosaic pattern. In the second figure, note that the low-attenuation areas of the lung have a diminished number and size of vessels compared with adjacent areas of higher attenuation. In patients with chronic pulmonary thromboembolism, this pattern reflects the diminished blood flow to areas of the lung distal to chronic emboli.

The vascular hallmark of chronic pulmonary thromboembolism is the presence of a mural thrombus. Chronic thrombus is typically adherent to the vascular wall, and it may contain foci of calcification. You may also observe an asymmetry in the size of the segmental pulmonary arteries of the lungs in patients with chronic pulmonary thromboembolism.

Notes

C A S E   1 1 7

Complete Lung Collapse Secondary to an Endobronchial Lesion (Lymphoma)

1. Postobstructive atelectasis from an endobronchial lesion.

2. Lung cancer, carcinoid tumor, hamartoma, mucoepidermoid tumor, lymphoma, lipoma, and metastases.

3. Gastric wall thickening.

4. Lymphoma and breast cancer.

Reference

Armstrong P: Neoplasms of the lungs, airways, and pleura. In: Armstrong P, Wilson AG, Dee P, Hansell DM, Eds: *Imaging of Diseases of the Chest*, second edition. St. Louis, Mosby, 1995, p 325.

Cross-Reference

Thoracic Radiology: THE REQUISITES, pp 40, 337, 374–380.

Comment

When you observe complete opacification of a hemithorax on a chest radiograph, the two most likely causes are complete atelectasis of a lung and a large pleural effusion. These entities can be readily differentiated by assessing the position of the mediastinum. When atelectasis is the primary abnormality, the mediastinum will be shifted toward the side of opacification. In contrast, when a large pleural effusion is present, the mediastinum will be shifted in the opposite direction. In cases of postobstructive atelectasis from an endobronchial lesion, you may also observe an endobronchial filling defect, as seen in the first figure.

Postobstructive atelectasis of an entire lung may occur secondary to a variety of causes. In the intensive care unit setting, you should consider an obstructing mucous plug or a malpositioned endotracheal tube (e.g., right mainstem bronchus intubation). In an outpatient setting, an obstructing neoplasm or a foreign body (more common in children than in adults) is the most likely etiology. The combination of an endobronchial lesion and gastric wall thickening may occur secondary to lymphoma or breast cancer. Although an endobronchial lesion is a rare manifestation of lymphoma, it is the best fit for the imaging findings in this young adult man.

Notes

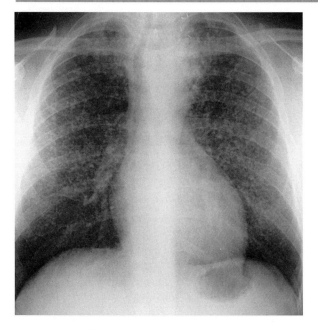
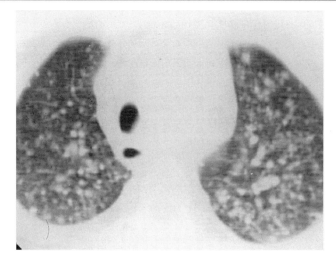

1. Name at least two neoplasms that may result in a fine nodular pattern of metastases.

2. Name at least three neoplasms that may result in calcified metastases.

3. Name at least two nonneoplastic causes of a diffuse, fine nodular pattern with calcification.

4. What is the most likely diagnosis in this case?

Metastatic Thyroid Carcinoma

1. Thyroid, melanoma, renal cell carcinoma, and adenocarcinomas (e.g., breast, pancreas).

2. Thyroid, breast, ovary, colon, sarcomas, and successfully treated metastases.

3. Healed varicella, healed histoplasmosis, silicosis.

4. Metastatic thyroid cancer.

Reference

Armstrong P: Neoplasms of the lungs, airways, and pleura. In: Armstrong P, Wilson AG, Dee P, Hansell DM, Eds: *Imaging of Diseases of the Chest*, second edition. St. Louis, Mosby, 1995, p 346.

Cross-Reference

Thoracic Radiology: THE REQUISITES, p 336.

Comment

The radiograph and CT image demonstrate a diffuse, fine nodular pattern of parenchymal opacities. The majority of nodules are 2 to 3 mm in diameter, although a few are slightly larger. The small nodules are well visualized on the radiograph because they are calcified.

Although there are a variety of causes of a fine nodular pattern, only a few entities result in calcified nodules. These entities include healed varicella, healed histoplasmosis, silicosis, and calcified metastases.

With the exception of osteosarcoma and chondrosarcoma, detectable calcification in metastases is unusual. A variety of mucinous and papillary neoplasms may rarely result in calcified metastases. Thyroid carcinoma is the most common cause of a fine nodular pattern of calcified metastases.

An important ancillary finding in this case is the presence of a superior mediastinal mass, with associated compression and deviation of the trachea. Such masses are usually related to the thyroid gland. In this patient, the mass represents thyroid carcinoma, and the calcified nodules are secondary to metastases.

Notes

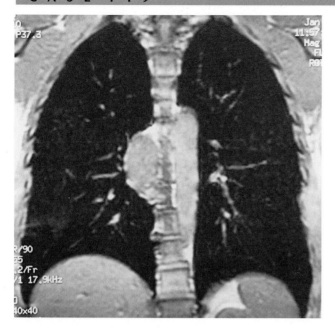
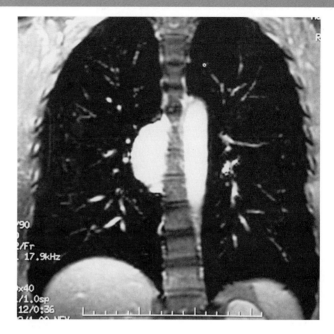
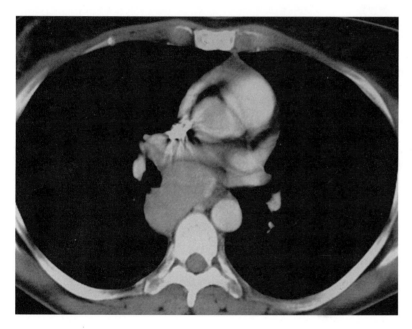

1. Name a benign cause of enhancing mediastinal lymph nodes.

2. What neoplasms are typically associated with enhancing mediastinal lymph nodes?

3. Which of the two subtypes of Castleman's disease is more common: hyaline vascular or plasma cell?

4. Which of the two forms is more commonly associated with clinical manifestations?

Castleman's Disease (Benign Lymph Node Hyperplasia)

1. Castleman's disease (benign lymph node hyperplasia) and sarcoidosis (rare).

2. Renal cell carcinoma, thyroid cancer, and small cell lung cancer.

3. Hyaline vascular.

4. Plasma cell.

Reference
Johkoh T, Müller NL, Ichikado K, et al: Intrathoracic multicentric Castleman disease: CT findings in 12 patients. *Radiology* 209:477–481, 1998.

Cross-Reference
Thoracic Radiology: THE REQUISITES, pp 440–441.

Comment
Pregadolinium and postgadolinium coronal MRIs in the first and second figures and a contrast-enhanced CT image in the third figure demonstrate an enhancing nodal mass in the subcarinal region that extends into the azygoesophageal recess. The identification of enhancing nodes significantly narrows the wide differential diagnosis of mediastinal lymph node enlargement. In a majority of cases, enhancing nodes are due to metastatic disease from hypervascular neoplasms such as renal cell or thyroid carcinoma. The most common benign etiology is Castleman's disease, the diagnosis in this case.

Castleman's disease, also referred to as benign lymph node hyperplasia, is an uncommon benign lymphoproliferative disorder. This disorder has been divided into two histologic subtypes: hyaline vascular and plasma cell. The hyaline vascular subtype is present in the vast majority (90%) of cases. This subtype is characterized by hyperplasia of lymphoid follicles with germinal center formation and the presence of numerous capillaries with hyalinized walls. It usually manifests as a solitary hilar or mediastinal enhancing nodal mass in asymptomatic patients.

The plasma cell subtype is characterized by the presence of mature plasma cells between the hyperplastic germinal centers and relatively few capillaries. This form is frequently associated with clinical symptoms, including fever, fatigue, anemia, polyclonal hypergammaglobulinemia, and bone marrow plasmacytosis. In contrast with the hyaline vascular subtype, bilateral hilar and multifocal mediastinal lymph node enlargement is commonly observed. Another differentiating feature is the relatively low level of enhancement of nodes observed in the plasma cell subtype compared with the marked enhancement of nodes in the hyaline vascular subtype.

Interestingly, the plasma cell subtype may also be associated with lymphocytic interstitial pneumonitis (LIP). Common CT imaging features of LIP include centrilobular nodules, cysts, and thickening of bronchovascular bundles and interlobular septa. Less frequent manifestations include ground-glass opacities, airspace consolidation, and bronchiectasis.

Notes

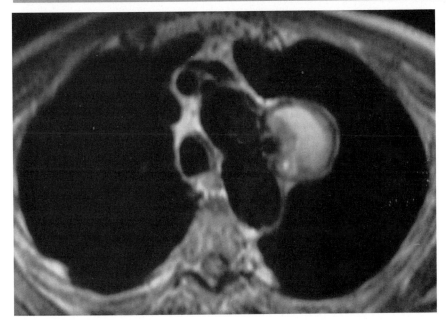

1. Name at least three substances that are associated with increased signal intensity on T1W MRI.

2. What is the normal appearance of flowing blood within vessels on spin-echo sequences?

3. If this mass is of vascular origin, how can you explain the presence of increased signal intensity?

4. Are spin-echo sequences associated with "black blood" or "white blood" imaging?

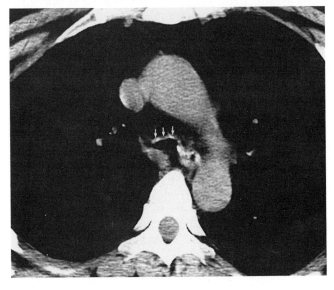 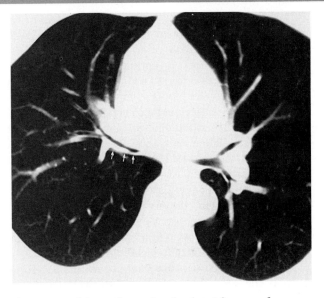

1. In addition to the abnormalities illustrated in these CT images, this patient also had evidence of auricular and nasal abnormalities. What is the most likely cause of airway narrowing?

2. Name at least three additional entities that may be associated with diffuse tracheobronchial narrowing.

3. Which one of these entities characteristically spares the posterior wall of the trachea?

4. Does relapsing polychondritis preferentially involve the proximal or distal airways?

Thrombosed Saccular Aortic Aneurysm

1. Fat, hemorrhage (methemoglobin), high protein content, gadolinium, and slow flow in vessels.

2. Signal void (black blood).

3. Thrombosis or slow flow.

4. Black blood.

Reference

Naidich DP, Webb WR, Müller NL, et al, Eds: Aorta, arch vessels, and great veins. In: *Computed Tomography and Magnetic Resonance of the Thorax*, third edition. Philadelphia, Lippincott-Raven, 1999, pp 508–516.

Cross-Reference

Thoracic Radiology: THE REQUISITES, pp 447–449.

Comment

The MRI demonstrates a middle mediastinal mass that contacts the lateral aspect of the aortic arch. Whenever you identify a mass immediately adjacent to the aorta, you should always consider an aneurysm. In most cases, the vascular nature of a mass can be readily confirmed by contrast-enhanced CT or MRI.

Vascular imaging with MR usually employs both black blood and white blood imaging techniques. Black blood imaging, as shown in this case, refers to spin-echo sequences. Such sequences result in signal void (black blood) from flowing blood within vascular structures. Although such techniques are excellent for demonstrating the anatomy of vascular structures, including vascular walls and luminal diameter, they are not ideal for assessing luminal flow. In contrast, white blood techniques are preferable for assessing luminal flow. There are a variety of white blood techniques, including cine gradient-echo (GRE), two-dimensional (2D) segmented time-of-flight, 2D gadolinium-enhanced rapid GRE imaging, and gadolinium-enhanced 3D angiography. These white blood techniques can readily differentiate slow flow from thrombus.

This case is challenging. Note the black blood appearance of the aorta in contrast with the increased signal within most of this paraaortic mass. It is important to be aware that slow flow within vascular structures may result in increased signal intensity on T1W images.

An important clue to the diagnosis of this paraaortic mass is the identification of a small, round focus of signal void medially, which connects with the adjacent aortic lumen. Thus, this mass represents a saccular aortic aneurysm. The high signal intensity within the majority of the mass can be explained by either extensive thrombosis or slow flow. A conventional thoracic aortogram confirmed the presence of a thrombosed saccular aortic aneurysm.

Notes

Relapsing Polychondritis

1. Relapsing polychondritis.

2. Tracheopathia osteochondroplastica, Wegener's granulomatosis, amyloidosis, sarcoidosis, and infection (papillomatosis, rhinosclerosis, tuberculosis).

3. Tracheopathia osteochondroplastica.

4. Proximal.

Reference

Shepard JAO: The bronchi: an imaging perspective. *J Thorac Imaging* 10:236–254, 1995.

Cross-Reference

Thoracic Radiology: THE REQUISITES, pp 349–361.

Comment

The CT images in this case demonstrate diffuse narrowing of the trachea (first figure) and bronchi (second figure), with associated thickening of the tracheal and bronchial walls *(arrows)*. As listed in Answer 2, there are a variety of causes of diffuse tracheobronchial narrowing.

Relapsing polychondritis is a rare inflammatory disease that affects cartilages of the ears, nose, upper respiratory tract, and joints. The etiology of this condition is uncertain, but it may be related to abnormal mucopolysaccharide metabolism or an autoimmune vasculitis. Recurrent bouts of inflammation result in fragmentation and subsequent fibrosis of cartilaginous structures. Auricular chondritis is the most common manifestation of this disorder, occurring in approximately 90% of patients. Respiratory tract involvement is seen in roughly 50% of patients and is the major cause of morbidity associated with this condition.

With regard to airway involvement, the larynx, trachea, and mainsteam bronchi are most commonly affected. Segmental and subsegmental bronchi are affected less frequently. Initially, airway narrowing results from mucosal edema. Later in the course of this condition, edema is replaced by granulation tissue and fibrosis. Airway involvement results in impaired clearance of secretions that may be complicated by recurrent respiratory infections and bronchiectasis.

Notes

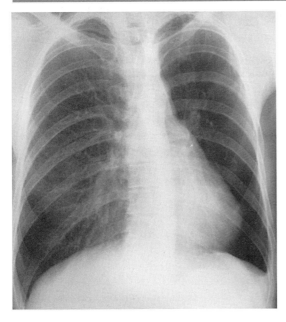

1. Name the syndrome characterized by a unilateral hyperlucent lung or lobe secondary to an obliterative bronchiolitis.

2. What is the cause of this syndrome?

3. What methods can be used to demonstrate air trapping in patients with this condition?

4. What airway abnormality is frequently demonstrated on CT scans of patients with this syndrome?

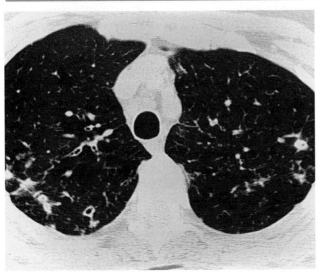 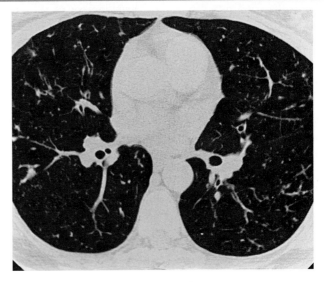

1. What is the most likely cause for the bronchiectasis and centrilobular nodules in this elderly woman who presents with a chronic cough?

2. Is this the classic form of *Mycobacterium avium* complex (MAC) infection?

3. Is bronchopulmonary MAC infection acquired by human-to-human transmission?

4. In older women with MAC infection, which lobes of the lungs are most frequently affected?

C A S E 1 2 2

Swyer-James Syndrome

1. Swyer-James syndrome.

2. Acute viral bronchiolitis in infancy or childhood.

3. Expiratory radiograph or CT and nuclear medicine ventilation scan.

4. Bronchiectasis.

Reference

Webb WR, Müller NL, Naidich DP: Diseases characterized primarily by decreased lung opacity, including cystic abnormalities, emphsyema, and bronchiectasis. In: *High-Resolution CT of the Lung*, second edition. Philadelphia, Lippincott-Raven, 1996, p 260.

Cross-Reference

Thoracic Radiology: THE REQUISITES, p 400.

Comment

The chest radiograph demonstrates hyperlucency of the left lung with associated reduced pulmonary vascularity, which is most marked in the left lower lobe. Also note the slightly reduced size of the left lung compared with the right lung.

The imaging findings are characteristic of Swyer-James syndrome, a variant of postinfectious obliterative bronchiolitis. This syndrome occurs secondary to an acute viral bronchiolitis in early infancy or early childhood that prevents the normal development of the affected lung. As shown in this case, the typical inspiratory radiograph findings include a unilateral hyperlucent lung or lobe with normal or reduced volume and reduced pulmonary vascularity. Expiratory radiographs (not shown) reveal air trapping.

High-resolution CT imaging features of Swyer-James syndrome include (1) areas of decreased lung attenuation with associated reduction in the number and size of vessels; (2) bronchiectasis; and (3) air trapping on expiratory images. Interestingly, although radiographic findings in patients with Swyer-James syndrome are typically unilateral, CT scanning often shows patchy areas of abnormality within the opposite lung as well.

Notes

C A S E 1 2 3

Mycobacterium avium Complex Infection

1. MAC infection.

2. No.

3. No.

4. Middle lobe and lingula.

Reference

Patz EF, Swensen SJ, Erasmus J: Pulmonary manifestations of nontuberculous *Mycobacterium. Radiol Clin North Am* 33:719–729, 1995.

Cross-Reference

Thoracic Radiology: THE REQUISITES, pp 121–122.

Comment

Nontuberculous mycobacterial (NTMB) infection is usually caused by MAC and *Mycobacterium kansasii*. These organisms are found in soil and water and demonstrate similar features.

NTMB affects two main groups of patients, who present with distinct demographic, clinical, and radiographic features. The first group consists primarily of older men with chronic obstructive pulmonary disease (COPD). Such patients present with the classic form of NTMB infection, which may occur secondary to either MAC or *M. kansasii*. Clinical symptoms are often insidious and include cough, hemoptysis, and constitutional symptoms. The imaging features are almost identical to reactivation TB and are characterized by slowly progressive fibronodular opacities that are often associated with cavitation. The apical and posterior segments of the upper lobes and the superior segments of the lower lobes are most commonly involved.

The second group of patients is composed of elderly women with MAC infection. Such patients are immunocompetent and do not have a history of COPD. They typically present with a chronic cough, but hemoptysis and constitutional symptoms are usually absent. The imaging features of MAC in this subgroup are best demonstrated by CT and include cylindrical bronchiectasis and multiple small (usually <5-mm diameter) lung nodules. Foci of ground-glass opacification and consolidation may be encountered in some cases. In contrast with the classic form, cavitation is uncommon in this subgroup. Although the distribution may be diffuse, the middle lobe and lingula are most commonly involved.

Because NTMB are common contaminants, a diagnosis requires (1) evidence of cavitation or progressive changes on radiographs (classic form); (2) at least two positive sputum cultures; or (3) evidence of mycobacteria on biopsy. Precise identification of the infecting organism is important for directing appropriate therapy.

Notes

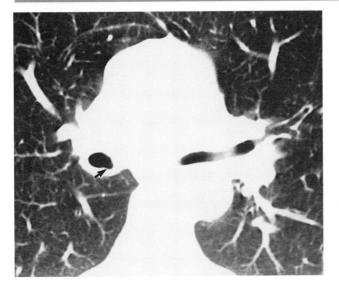
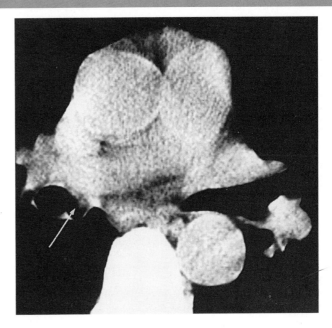

1. What is the term used to describe this bronchial abnormality?
2. Is this a congenital or an acquired condition?
3. From what portion of the airway does it arise?
4. Name at least one symptom associated with this condition.

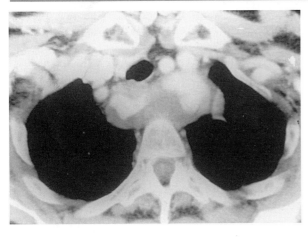
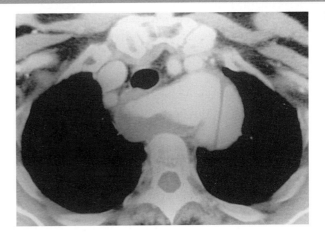

1. What congenital vascular abnormality is present?
2. What is the prevalence of this anomaly?
3. What is the term used to describe the swallowing difficulty associated with this anomaly?
4. What acquired aortic abnormality is also present in this case?

Cardiac Bronchus

1. Cardiac bronchus.

2. Congenital.

3. Bronchus intermedius.

4. Recurrent infections, hemoptysis, cough, and dyspnea.

Reference

McGuinness G, Naidich DP, Garay SM, et al: Accessory cardiac bronchus: CT features and clinical significance. *Radiology* 189:563–566, 1993.

Cross-Reference

None.

Comment

The CT images in this case demonstrate an anomalous blind-ending diverticulum *(arrows)* arising from the medial wall of the bronchus intermedius. This structure represents a cardiac bronchus, the only known true supernumerary anomalous bronchus. Other anomalies of the airway involve either a normal number of bronchi with ectopic locations (e.g., aberrant tracheal bronchus) or an absence of bronchi (e.g., bronchial atresia).

The cardiac bronchus always arises from the same location—from the medial wall of the bronchus intermedius, above the origin of the superior segment bronchus. It is directed caudally toward the mediastinum. For this reason, it has been coined the "cardiac" bronchus.

Its length varies from a small, blind-ending pouch (such as in this case) to a longer branching structure. The longer configuration may be associated with rudimentary alveolar tissue in some cases. The cardiac bronchus is lined by endobronchial mucosa and contains cartilaginous rings within its walls.

This anomaly is usually incidentally discovered in asymptomatic patients. However, because a cardiac bronchus may serve as a reservoir for infectious material, affected patients may present with recurrent respiratory infections. Resultant inflammation and hypervascularity may also result in hemoptysis. Surgical excision is recommended for symptomatic patients.

Notes

Aberrant Right Subclavian Artery With Aortic Dissection

1. Aberrant right subclavian artery.

2. Approximately 1%.

3. Dysphagia lusoria.

4. Aortic dissection.

Reference

Freed K, Low VHS: The aberrant subclavian artery. *AJR Am J Roentgenol* 166:481–484, 1997.

Cross-Reference

Thoracic Radiology: THE REQUISITES, pp 443–445.

Comment

An aberrant right subclavian artery (ARSA) is the most common intrathoracic major arterial anomaly, with an incidence of approximately 1%. The ARSA arises as the last branch of the aortic arch and courses cephalad obliquely from left to right behind the trachea and esophagus. An aortic diverticulum, the diverticulum of Kommerell, may be present at the origin of this vessel.

In most patients, the anomaly is asymptomatic and discovered incidentally. A small minority of patients may develop difficulty in swallowing secondary to esophageal compression.

On chest radiography, you may observe the ARSA as an oblique opacity coursing superiorly from left to right, beginning at the level of the aortic arch. On barium swallow examinations, you may observe a characteristic oblique indentation on the posterior wall of the esophagus. An ARSA is easily identified on cross-sectional imaging studies such as the CT images in the figures. On such studies, the ARSA appears as a tubular structure arising from the aortic arch and coursing cephalad obliquely behind the trachea and esophagus. Aneurysmal dilation of the proximal portion of the ARSA is observed in roughly 10% of cases.

This case also demonstrates the presence of an aortic dissection. Note the presence of an intimal flap, which appears as a linear soft tissue density within the contrast-opacified vessels. Aortic dissection is characterized by a tear in the intima of the aortic wall, followed by separation of the tunica media. This process results in the creation of two channels for the passage of blood: a true and a false lumen.

Once you have identified an aortic dissection, it is important to determine its precise extent. Involvement of the ascending aorta (Stanford type A) requires surgical therapy. Extension of the dissection into the great vessels is an important preoperative finding. In contrast, isolated descending aortic dissections (Stanford type B) are generally managed medically.

Notes

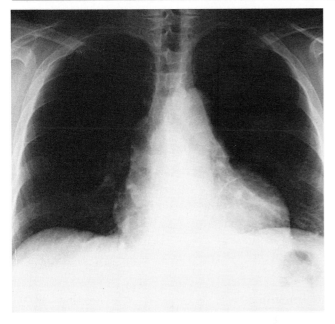
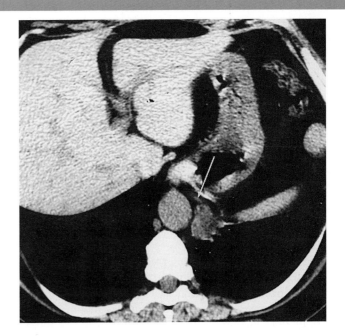

1. What is the most common source of arterial blood supply for a sequestration?

2. Which form of sequestration is more common, intralobar or extralobar?

3. Are sequestrations more common in the left or the right lung?

4. What is the usual drainage site for an intralobar sequestration?

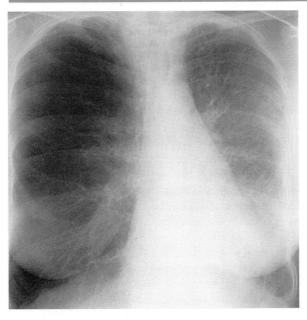
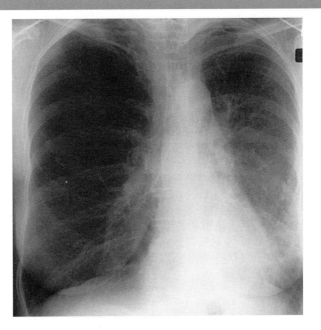

1. This patient is status post transplantation of the left lung 2 weeks prior to the date of these radiographs, which were obtained 2 days apart. Considering this time interval, is reperfusion edema (reimplantation response) a likely diagnosis?

2. Are pleural effusions a common finding in patients with acute rejection?

3. Does a normal chest radiograph exclude the presence of acute rejection?

4. On what basis is a diagnosis of acute rejection typically made?

CASE 126

Intralobar Sequestration

1. Descending thoracic aorta.

2. Intralobar.

3. Left.

4. Inferior pulmonary vein.

Reference

Ellis K: Developmental abnormalities in the systemic blood supply to the lung. *AJR Am J Roentgenol* 156:669–679, 1991.

Cross-Reference

Thoracic Radiology: THE REQUISITES, pp 77–79.

Comment

The chest radiograph demonstrates a focal opacity in the posterior basal segment of the left lower lobe, which obscures a portion of the descending thoracic aortic interface and medial left hemidiaphragm. The CT image reveals a discrete soft tissue density mass that contains two tiny cystic foci. Note the presence of an adjacent tubular structure *(arrow)*, which represents a systemic artery from the descending thoracic aorta. The imaging findings are consistent with a sequestration, which refers to an area of aberrant lung tissue that has no normal connection with the bronchial tree or pulmonary arteries and is supplied by a systemic artery.

Sequestrations are classified as either intralobar (contained within the substance of the lung) or extralobar (contained within its own pleural envelope). Intralobar sequestration is the most common type. Affected patients may be asymptomatic or may present with a history of recurrent pulmonary infections. The posterior basal segment is the most common location, and the left lung is affected twice as often as the right lung. Intralobar sequestrations may appear radiographically as a solid mass, a focal area of consolidation, or a cystic or multicystic lesion. The identification of a systemic arterial supply confirms the diagnosis. A systemic artery is usually visible on either contrast-enhanced CT or MRI. Failure to detect such a vessel does not exclude the diagnosis, however, and angiography may be required for definitive diagnosis in some cases.

In contrast with intralobar sequestration, the extralobar variety usually presents during infancy. The typical radiographic appearance is a well-defined, solitary mass in close proximity to the posteromedial aspect of the hemidiaphragm. Less frequent sites of involvement include mediastinal and subdiaphragmatic locations. Approximately 90% of cases are in the left hemithorax. The arterial supply may arise from single or multiple systemic arteries. Extralobar sequestration is associated with systemic venous drainage, usually to the azygos system.

Notes

CASE 127

Acute Rejection Following Lung Transplantation

1. No.

2. Yes.

3. No.

4. Histologic analysis of transbronchial biopsy specimens.

Reference

Erasmus JJ, McAdams HP, Tapson VF, et al: Radiologic issues in lung transplantation for end-stage pulmonary disease. *AJR Am J Roentgenol* 169:69–78, 1997.

Cross-Reference

None.

Comment

Lung transplantation is a potentially life-saving therapeutic option for certain patients with end-stage pulmonary disease. Because of the limited supply of donor lungs, single rather than double-lung transplantation is usually performed. Single-lung transplantation is also technically easier to perform and has a slightly lower morbidity and mortality than double-lung transplantation. Most pulmonary disorders, including various causes of pulmonary fibrosis and emphysema, can be successfully managed with single-lung transplantation. Exceptions are disorders such as cystic fibrosis that are associated with chronically infected lungs. Such patients require double-lung transplantation. Recently, transplantation of lobes from living-related donors has also been performed in patients with cystic fibrosis.

Early pulmonary postoperative complications of lung transplantation include reperfusion edema, acute rejection, and infection. Reperfusion edema, also referred to as reimplantation response, is caused by increased capillary permeability and occurs in the vast majority of transplanted lungs. It has a characteristic time course, usually beginning in the first 24 hours, peaking between 1 and 5 days, and resolving within approximately 10 days following transplantation. Acute rejection is a common complication within the first 3 months following transplantation. The first episode usually occurs in the first 5 to 10 days following surgery. Note that reperfusion edema begins earlier and peaks before this time. Infection is the most common pulmonary complication following transplantation. The type of organism varies depending on the time interval from surgery. In the first month, bacterial infections are most common. After the first month, atypical infections such as cytomegalovirus are most common.

Notes

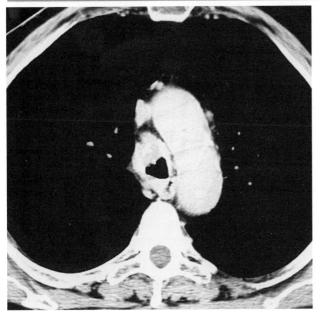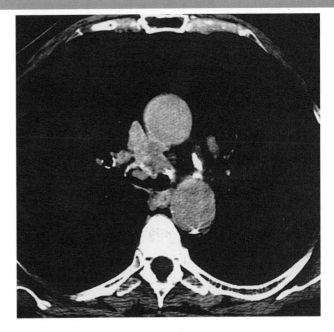

1. What is the most likely mechanism for involvement of the airways by TB in this case?

2. Are the imaging features suggestive of the hyperplastic or fibrostenotic stage of TB airway involvement?

3. Is the hyperplastic form of tuberculous airways disease potentially reversible with therapy?

4. Are these imaging findings specific for an infectious process?

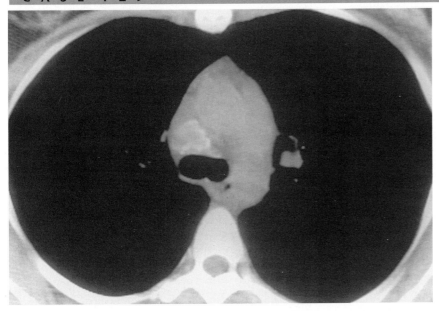

1. Name two common infectious causes of mediastinal lymph node enlargement in patients with human immunodeficiency virus (HIV) infection.

2. Name two acquired immunodeficiency syndrome (AIDS)-related neoplasms that may result in mediastinal lymph node enlargement.

3. On the non-contrast CT image, what does the increased attenuation within the enlarged precarinal lymph node represent?

4. What opportunistic infection is associated with calcified lymph nodes?

Tuberculosis Involving the Airways

1. Direct invasion from adjacent mediastinal lymph nodes.

2. Hyperplastic.

3. Yes.

4. No—neoplasm should be excluded.

Reference

Moon WK, Mim J, Yeon KM, Han MC: Tuberculosis of the central airways: CT findings of active and fibrotic disease. *AJR Am J Roentgenol* 169:648-653, 1997.

Cross-Reference

Thoracic Radiology: THE REQUISITES, p 358.

Comment

Airway involvement in patients with TB may result from several mechanisms: (1) direct contact of the airway mucosa with infected secretions; (2) submucosal spread of infection through the lymphatics from infected lymph nodes or lung; and (3) direct invasion of the airway by adjacent lymph nodes.

There are two stages of tracheobronchial involvement by TB. The first stage is characterized by hyperplastic changes. During this stage, tubercles form in the submucosal layer and are accompanied by ulceration and necrosis of the airway wall. The affected airway walls appear irregularly thickened with variable degrees of luminal narrowing. Hilar and mediastinal lymph node enlargement are commonly observed and frequently demonstrate peripheral enhancement with central low attenuation. Cavitary lung lesions may occasionally be seen within the lobes drained by the affected bronchi.

In the first figure, note the presence of irregular thickening of the anterior and lateral wall of the trachea, with eccentric luminal narrowing. In the second figure, there is irregular, lobulated thickening of the anterior wall of the airway with polypoid intraluminal extension. The contiguity of the airway disease with adjacent mediastinal lymph nodes suggests that the airway involvement is due to direct invasion by tuberculous lymph nodes.

The second stage is characterized by fibrostenotic features. In this stage, the bronchi are typically smoothly narrowed. The fibrostenotic phase can be complicated by postobstructive collapse.

In a study of 41 patients with TB of the airway, patients with a hyperplastic stage of TB demonstrated irregular and thick-walled airways, a pattern frequently reversible with medical therapy. In contrast, patients with fibrotic disease generally demonstrated smooth narrowing of the airways and minimal wall thickening, a pattern not reversible with medical therapy.

Notes

Calcified Mediastinal Lymph Nodes Secondary to Disseminated *Pneumocystis carinii* Pneumonia

1. Mycobacterial (TB and NTMB) and fungal infections.

2. Kaposi's sarcoma and lymphoma.

3. Calcification.

4. Disseminated *Pneumocystis carinii* pneumonia (PCP).

Reference

Boiselle PM, Crans CA Jr, Kaplan MA: The changing face of *Pneumocystis carinii* pneumonia in AIDS patients. *AJR Am J Roentgenol* 172:1301-1309, 1999.

Cross-Reference

Thoracic Radiology: THE REQUISITES, pp 142-149.

Comment

Mediastinal lymph node enlargement in patients with HIV infection is most commonly caused by TB or Kaposi's sarcoma. Less common causes include fungal infections, atypical mycobacterial infection (e.g., MAC), and lymphoma.

CT is helpful for identifying and characterizing enlarged mediastinal lymph nodes. For example, in an HIV-positive patient, the presence of low-density lymph nodes with peripheral rim enhancement is characteristic of mycobacterial or fungal infections rather than a neoplastic process.

In this case, there is an enlarged precarinal lymph node with peripheral rim calcification and some subtle intranodal calcifications. Although PCP is an uncommon cause of nodal enlargement in HIV-positive patients, the disseminated form of this infection may result in calcified nodes in the mediastinum and abdomen. Such nodes typically demonstrate stippled or punctate internal calcifications and peripheral, "rim-like" calcifications. Additional sites of calcification may include the liver, kidneys, spleen, and pancreas. In the proper clinical setting, the appearance is characteristic of disseminated PCP. A disseminated mycobacterial infection may result in a similar appearance.

The disseminated form of PCP is often, but not always, associated with aerosolized pentamidine use. In patients receiving this prophylactic agent, the drug reaches sufficient concentrations in the lungs to suppress pulmonary infection, but the level of systemic concentration may be too low to prevent disseminated infection. Because aerosolized pentamidine has been largely replaced by more effective agents (such as trimethoprim-sulfamethoxazole [Bactrim]), the disseminated form of PCP is uncommonly encountered today.

Notes

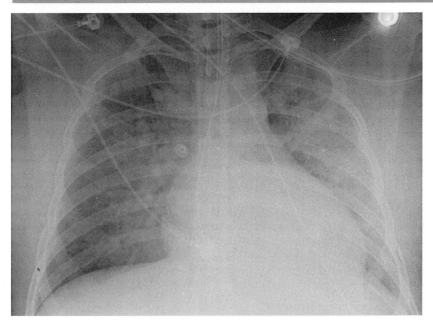

1. Name at least one cardiogenic cause of pulmonary edema associated with pregnancy.
2. Name at least one noncardiogenic cause of pulmonary edema associated with pregnancy.
3. Is pregnancy associated with an increased prevalence of pulmonary thromboembolic disease?
4. Why are pregnant patients at increased risk for community-acquired pneumonias?

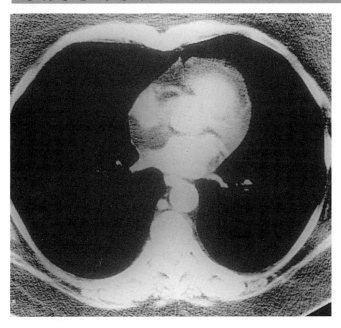

1. What term is used to describe the fat-attenuation mass located in the interatrial septum in the figure?
2. Is this a benign or malignant process?
3. In what percentage of cases is this process associated with diffuse mediastinal lipomatosis?
4. Does lipomatous hypertrophy of the interatrial septum (LHIS) enhance following intravenous contrast administration?

CASE 130

Pregnancy Complicated by Pulmonary Edema Secondary to Preeclampsia

1. Peripartum cardiomyopathy and hypertension (preeclampsia).

2. Tocolytic therapy and amniotic fluid embolism.

3. Yes.

4. Pregnancy is associated with a depression in cell-mediated immunity.

Reference

Fidler JL, Patz EF, Ravin CE: Cardiopulmonary complications of pregnancy: radiographic findings. *AJR Am J Roentgenol* 161:937–941, 1993.

Cross-Reference

None.

Comment

Pregnancy is normally associated with a variety of cardiopulmonary physiologic changes. Maternal blood volume and cardiac output increase by roughly 45% by midpregnancy. These changes are associated with increased pulmonary vascularity and progressive left ventricular dilation and mild hypertrophy.

There are a variety of cardiopulmonary complications of pregnancy, including cardiogenic and noncardiogenic pulmonary edema, pulmonary thromboembolism, aspiration pneumonitis, and pneumonia. Other rare complications include metastatic disease from gestational trophoblastic neoplasm, pneumothorax, and pneumomediastinum.

The patient in this case developed preeclampsia during her third trimester of pregnancy that was complicated by pulmonary edema. Preeclampsia is characterized by the development of hypertension, proteinuria, and edema after 24 weeks' gestation. *Eclampsia* refers to the development of seizures. In patients with preeclampsia, hypertension may become severe enough to produce acute cardiac failure. Radiographs typically show pulmonary edema with a variable heart size. In this patient, the pulmonary edema was asymmetric, reflecting gravitational dependency of pulmonary edema due to the patient's preference for lying on her left side. Another cardiogenic cause of pulmonary edema is peripartum cardiomyopathy, which occurs in the last month of pregnancy or in the first 6 months following delivery. Radiographs demonstrate marked cardiac enlargement that may be accompanied by pulmonary edema.

Notes

CASE 131

Lipomatous Hypertrophy of the Interatrial Septum

1. LHIS.

2. Benign.

3. Approximately 50%.

4. No.

Reference

Meaney JF, Kazerooni EA, Jamadar DA, Korobkin M: CT appearance of lipomatous hypertrophy of the interatrial septum. *AJR Am J Roentgenol* 168:1081–1084, 1997.

Cross-Reference

None.

Comment

LHIS refers to the presence of a fat-attenuation interatrial mass. LHIS is usually incidentally detected on CT scans of asymptomatic patients. An association with atrial arrhthymias has been reported in some cases and is thought to occur secondary to disruption of septal conduction pathways.

Pathologically, LHIS demonstrates multiloculated, granular lipocytes within the interatrial septum. These lipocytes are the morphologic cells found in fetal or brown fat.

The typical CT appearance is a nonenhancing, smoothly marginated, dumbbell-shaped, homogeneous, fat-attenuation mass that is usually confined to the interatrial septum.

Notes

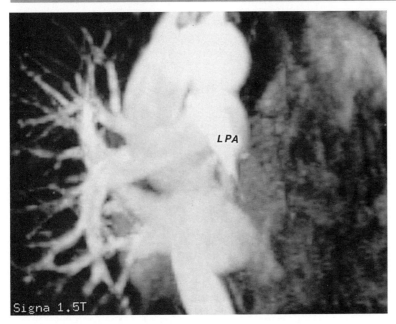

1. What is the striking abnormality on this MR angiogram?

2. Is a unilateral central pulmonary embolus a common distribution of acute pulmonary thromboembolism?

3. What is the radiographic sign used to describe oligemia distal to an obstructing embolus?

4. On MRI, how can you differentiate a pulmonary artery sarcoma from an acute thrombus?

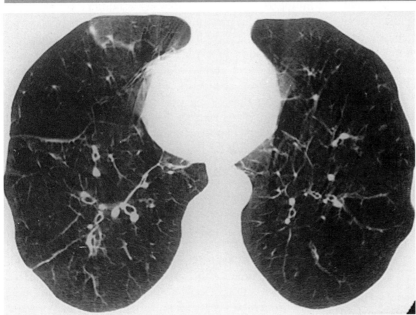

1. What disorder is most closely associated with a basilar distribution of panlobular emphysema?

2. Is there any association between this entity and bronchiectasis?

3. How is this disorder inherited?

4. Name an extrathoracic complication of this disorder.

CASE 132

Massive Unilateral Pulmonary Embolus

1. Abrupt cutoff of the left main pulmonary artery (LPA).

2. No.

3. Westermark's sign.

4. Only a pulmonary artery sarcoma enhances with gadolinium.

Reference

Weinreb JC, Davis SD, Berkman YM, Isom W, Naidich DP: Pulmonary artery sarcoma: evaluation using Gd-DTPA. *J Comp Assist Tomogr* 14:647–650, 1990.

Cross-Reference

Thoracic Radiology: THE REQUISITES, pp 412–419.

Comment

The MR angiogram demonstrates a normal appearance of the pulmonary vasculature of the right lung and complete absence of pulmonary vasculature within the left lung. Note the abrupt cutoff of the LPA due to an acute embolus.

A unilateral, completely obstructing embolus is an uncommon manifestation of acute pulmonary thromboembolism. In fact, when confronted with a nuclear medicine ventilation-perfusion scan that demonstrates a unilateral absence of perfusion, you should first consider nonthromboembolic causes such as mediastinal and hilar masses, ascending aortic aneurysm and dissection, pulmonary artery hypoplasia and agenesis, and pulmonary artery sarcoma and pneumonectomy. In this patient, the MRI examination revealed an obstructing, nonenhancing intrinsic filling defect in the LPA, consistent with an acute pulmonary embolus.

Preliminary investigations have shown that MR angiography is highly accurate in the diagnosis of pulmonary emboli. To date, however, CT has played a larger role in this setting. This is probably due to the wider availability and lower cost of CT compared with MRI. Moreover, CT is superior to MR in imaging the lung parenchyma and often reveals an alternative diagnosis for patients without evidence of acute pulmonary thromboembolism. Advantages of MRI compared with CT include a lack of ionizing radiation and an absence of iodinated contrast material.

Notes

CASE 133

Alpha₁-Antitrypsin Deficiency

1. Alpha₁-antitrypsin (AAT) deficiency.

2. Yes.

3. Autosomal recessive.

4. Cirrhosis.

Reference

King MA, Stone JA, Diaz PT, et al: Alpha₁-antitrypsin deficiency: evaluation of bronchiectasis with CT. *Radiology* 199:137–141, 1996.

Cross-Reference

Thoracic Radiology: THE REQUISITES, pp 291–293.

Comment

The CT image demonstrates diffuse panlobular emphysema in the lower lung zones. The upper lobes (not shown) were relatively spared of this process. Panlobular emphysema is characterized by fewer and smaller-than-normal pulmonary vessels. This appearance has been described as a "simplification of normal lung architecture." AAT deficiency, the diagnosis in this case, is characterized by a basilar distribution of panlobular emphysema.

AAT deficiency also referred to as alpha₁-protease inhibitor deficiency, is an inherited disorder that is characterized by abnormally low levels of alpha₁-protease inhibitor. This protein inhibits a number of lysosomal proteases and prevents the damaging effects of elastases released by macrophages and neutrophils. Because the administration of elastase has been shown to produce emphysema in animal models, it is not surprising that patients with reduced levels of protease inhibitors are at risk for developing this complication. Patients who are homozygous for this disorder have a very low level (roughly 20% of normal) of alpha₁-protease inhibitor and are at high risk for developing emphysema. This risk is increased by cigarette smoking.

Interestingly, patients with AAT deficiency have a high prevalence of bronchiectasis, which has been reported in approximately 40% of cases. In the figure, note the presence of bronchial wall thickening and dilation, which is most pronounced in the right lower lobe. The mechanism by which bronchiectasis develops in these patients is uncertain. It has been hypothesized that destruction of elastic fibers in the walls of bronchi and bronchioles plays an important role in this process.

Notes

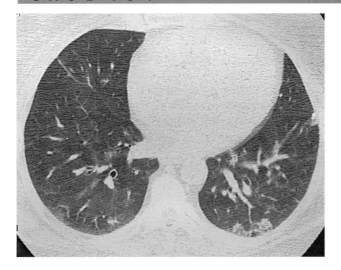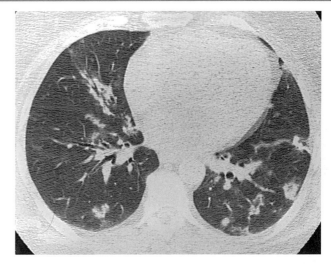

1. What is the predominant distribution of the parenchymal opacities shown in these CT images?

2. In contrast, what is the distribution of the focal right middle lobe consolidation shown in the second image?

3. Name at least three entities that typically present with a peripheral pattern of consolidation.

4. Which of these entities frequently demonstrates both peripheral and peribronchovascular foci of consolidation on CT imaging?

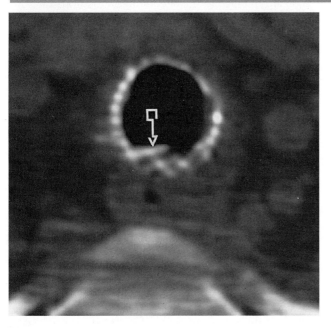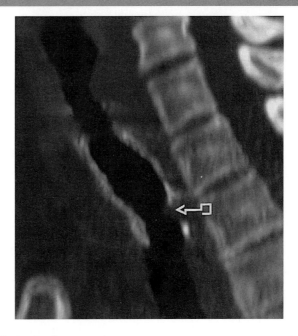

1. Name at least four indications for tracheobronchial stent placement.

2. List at least four potential complications of airway stent placement.

3. What complication is evident in this case?

4. Are airway stents easily removable?

Bronchiolitis Obliterans Organizing Pneumonia

1. Peripheral.

2. Peribronchovascular.

3. Bronchiolitis obliterans organizing pneumonia (BOOP), Löffler's syndrome, chronic eosinophilic pneumonia, pulmonary infarcts, and vasculitides.

4. BOOP.

Reference

Webb WR, Müller NL, Naidich DP: *High-Resolution CT of the Lung*, second edition. Philadelphia, Lippincott-Raven, 1996, pp 206–210.

Cross-Reference

Thoracic Radiology: THE REQUISITES, pp 225–226.

Comment

BOOP is characterized pathologically by the presence of granulation tissue polyps within bronchioles that extend more peripherally into the alveolar ducts with patchy areas of organizing pneumonia. The latter is the predominant feature of BOOP.

Although most cases are idiopathic, BOOP-like reactions have been described in association with a number of entities, including pulmonary infection, drug reactions, collagen-vascular disorders, and vasculitides.

Affected patients typically present clinically with a nonproductive cough. Associated symptoms may include dyspnea, malaise, and low-grade fever. The majority of cases respond to steroids and have a favorable prognosis. However, some patients relapse following cessation of therapy. Interestingly, relapse usually results in the reappearance of pulmonary opacities in the same distribution as the original presentation.

Radiographic findings consist primarily of patchy, nonsegmental, unilateral or bilateral foci of consolidation. The characteristic peripheral distribution of consolidation associated with BOOP may not be readily apparent on chest radiographs and is seen more frequently on CT scans.

Characteristic HRCT imaging features include patchy bilateral airspace consolidation with a peripheral, subpleural distribution. More recently, a peribronchovascular distribution has been described as a relatively frequent manifestation, often in association with foci of peripheral consolidation. Poorly defined lung nodules may also be observed and are often peribronchiolar in distribution. Thus, the presence of peripheral and peribronchovascular consolidation with associated small lung nodules in this case is most suggestive of BOOP. Less frequently observed findings associated with BOOP include bronchial wall thickening and bronchial dilation.

Notes

Fractured Tracheal Stent

1. Anastomotic narrowing following lung transplantation; palliative treatment of unresectable malignancy involving the trachea or bronchi; congenital or acquired tracheal stenosis; tracheobronchomalacia; external tracheal compression; and tracheal narrowing due to inflammatory or infectious etiologies.

2. Airway inflammation; stent migration; airway erosion; stent fracture; stent collapse; and tracheoesophageal fistula.

3. Stent fracture.

4. No.

Reference

Lehman JD, Gordon RL, Kerlan RK, et al: Expandable metallic stents in benign tracheobronchial obstruction. *J Thorac Imaging* 13:105–115, 1998.

Cross-Reference

None.

Comment

The axial CT image in the first figure and the 2D sagittal reformatted image in the second figure demonstrate the presence of a tracheal stent within the lower cervical portion of the trachea. Note the presence of focal stent fracture and disruption posteriorly *(arrows)*. This patient underwent stent placement for tracheal stenosis. She subsequently presented with evidence of wire fragments in her sputum, prompting this CT examination.

Expandable metallic stents are increasingly employed in the treatment of a variety of airway abnormalities. Once placed into the airway, metallic stents become incorporated into the bronchial wall or epithelialized, limiting potential migration and permitting ciliary activity to continue.

Prior to the advent of airway stenting, the treatment of tracheal stenosis was limited to surgical therapy. Surgical treatment of tracheal abnormalities with end-to-end reanastomosis is possible only when there is sufficient length of the airway. Stenting is not limited by this factor and thus provides an additional therapeutic option for many patients who are not surgical candidates.

One of the most important indications for placement of an airway stent is the presence of an unresectable malignancy involving the trachea or bronchi. In such patients, stents are usually used for palliation.

Prior to stent placement, CT accurately depicts the number and length of airway stenoses. Following placement of a stent, CT is an ideal modality for assessing for complications such as stent migration, stent fracture, and airway inflammation.

Notes

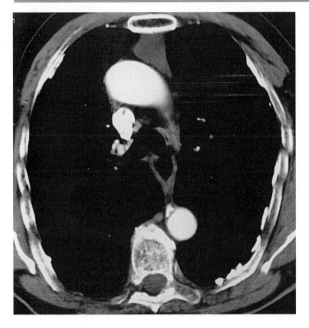 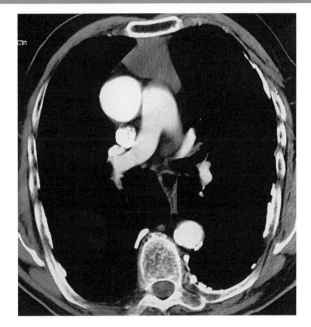

1. What is the most likely cause of this completely cystic anterior mediastinal mass?

2. Name at least two etiologies for an anterior mediastinal mass that contains solid and cystic elements.

3. What is the most common cause of a thymic mass?

4. If a thymic cyst has been complicated by hemorrhage, how would you expect it to appear on T1W MRI?

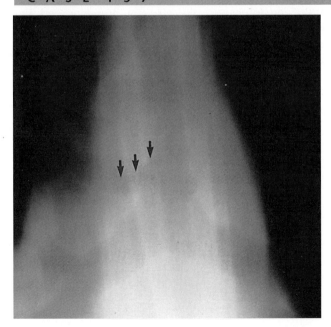

1. What congenital airway abnormality is evident on the tomogram image?

2. What portion of the lung does this anomalous bronchus usually supply?

3. Are patients with this finding usually symptomatic?

4. What potential complication can occur following intubation of a patient with this abnormality?

C A S E 1 3 6

Thymic Cyst

1. Thymic cyst.

2. Thymoma, Hodgkin's disease, and germ cell neoplasms.

3. Thymoma.

4. Bright (hemorrhage results in increased signal on T1W images as a result of the T1 shortening effect of methemoglobin).

Reference

Fraser RS, Colman N, Müller NL, Paré PD: Masses situated predominantly in the anterior mediastinal compartment. In: *Fraser and Paré's Diagnosis of Diseases of the Chest*, fourth edition. Philadelphia, WB Saunders, 1999, pp 2882–2884.

Cross-Reference

Thoracic Radiology: THE REQUISITES, p 435.

Comment

Thymic cysts are an uncommon cause of an anterior mediastinal mass. They may be congenital or acquired. Congenital cysts are probably derived from remnants of the fetal thymopharyngeal duct. Acquired cysts may develop following radiation therapy for Hodgkin's disease. Less commonly, they may occur following thoracic surgery or chemotherapy for a malignant neoplasm. An association with HIV infection has also been reported.

On imaging studies, a thymic cyst typically appears as a well-defined, cystic mass with an imperceptible wall. In a minority of cases, curvilinear calcifications may be identified within the wall of thymic cysts. On CT, thymic cysts typically demonstrate fluid attenuation. On MRI, thymic cysts usually demonstrate low signal intensity on T1W images and increased signal intensity on T2W images. However, the appearance may vary if the cyst has been complicated by hemorrhage or infection. The imaging features in this case are typical of an uncomplicated thymic cyst. Incidentally noted are numerous calcified pleural plaques, consistent with prior asbestos exposure.

When you identify an anterior mediastinal mass with solid and cystic components, you should consider the possibility of a solid anterior mediastinal mass that has undergone cystic necrosis. For example, thymoma and Hodgkin's lymphoma may contain cystic areas, occasionally associated with a relatively small amount of neoplastic tissue. Germ cell neoplasms such as mature teratomas frequently contain cystic components intermixed with solid elements. The identification of cystic elements in conjunction with fat and/or calcium should suggest this diagnosis.

Notes

C A S E 1 3 7

Tracheal Bronchus

1. Tracheal bronchus.

2. Right upper lobe (apical segment or entire lobe).

3. No.

4. Atelectasis of the portion of the lung supplied by the anomalous bronchus.

Reference

Wilson AG: Diseases of the airways. In: Armstrong P, Wilson AG, Dee P, Hansell DM, Eds: *Imaging of Diseases of the Chest*, second edition. St. Louis, Mosby, 1995, pp 826–828.

Cross-Reference

Thoracic Radiology: THE REQUISITES, pp 69, 71.

Comment

The tomogram demonstrates an anomalous bronchus (*arrows*) arising from the right lateral wall of the trachea, proximal to the origin of the right mainstem bronchus. The term *tracheal bronchus* has been used to describe this congenital bronchial anomaly, which may supply the apical segment of the right upper lobe or the entire right upper lobe.

Affected patients are usually asymptomatic. In a minority of cases, the bronchial orifice is narrow, which may lead to recurrent pneumonias and bronchiectasis. Following intubation, the aberrant bronchus may become occluded by the endotracheal tube balloon cuff, resulting in atelectasis within the corresponding segment or lobe that is supplied by the aberrant bronchus.

Notes

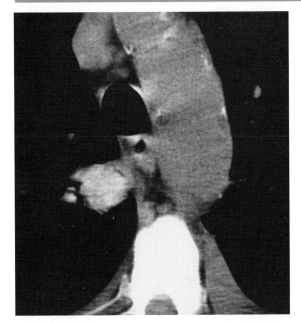
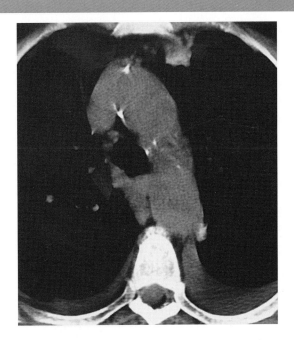
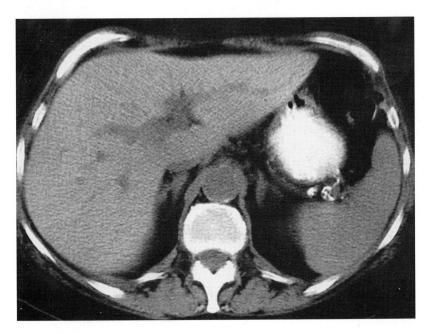

1. What is striking about these pulmonary nodules on this non-contrast CT?
2. Considering the presence of a hyperdense liver, what is the most likely etiology for these nodules?
3. What disorder is amiodarone used to treat?
4. What percentage of patients treated with amiodarone develop pulmonary toxicity?

Amiodarone Drug Toxicity

1. High attenuation.

2. Amiodarone toxicity.

3. Arrhythmias.

4. Approximately 5% to 20%.

Reference
Aronchick JM, Gefter WB: Drug-induced pulmonary disorders. *Semin Roentgenol* 30:18–34, 1995.

Cross-Reference
Thoracic Radiology: THE REQUISITES, pp 275, 276.

Comment
The non-contrast CT images presented in this case demonstrate several small pulmonary nodules with a subpleural distribution. Note the high attenuation of these lesions, a finding that is characteristic of lung toxicity due to amiodarone, a triiodinated compound that is used to treat cardiac arrhythmias. Pulmonary toxicity occurs in 5% to 20% of patients treated with amiodarone and is dose related.

There are two distinct clinical presentations of amiodarone toxicity. The most common presentation is a subacute onset of dyspnea, nonproductive cough, and weight loss. Radiographs typically reveal a diffuse linear pattern. A less common presentation (observed in approximately one third of patients) is characterized by an acute onset of symptoms that mimic an infectious pneumonitis. Radiographs of these patients typically demonstrate patchy alveolar opacities with a peripheral distribution. CT scans in these patients typically reveal high-attenuation foci of parenchymal opacification, with attenuation values ranging from approximately 80 to 175 Hounsfield units. This appearance reflects the high concentration of amiodarone, a triiodinated agent, within these regions of lung parenchyma.

Note the high attenuation of the liver in the second figure, a common finding in patients treated with amiodarone. Thus, the combination of high-attenuation focal parenchymal opacities and a high-attenuation liver is highly suggestive of amiodarone pulmonary toxicity. Prompt recognition is important, because amiodarone pulmonary toxicity is frequently reversible after withdrawal of the drug. Although clinical symptoms usually resolve within 2 to 4 weeks of drug withdrawal, chest radiographic abnormalities typically clear more slowly, in approximately 3 months.

Notes

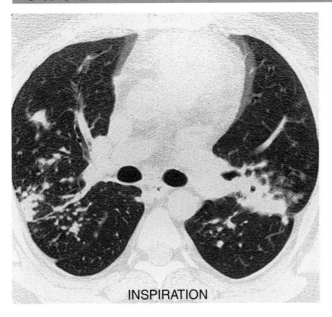

INSPIRATION

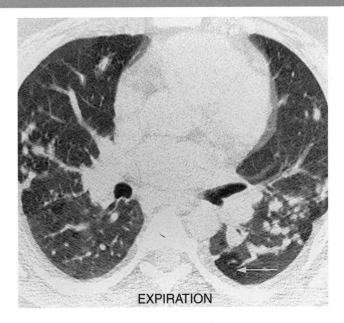

EXPIRATION

1. What is the predominant distribution of nodules shown in these high-resolution CT images?

2. Name at least three entities that can be associated with this distribution.

3. Which of these entities is frequently associated with symmetric hilar lymph node enlargement?

4. Is air trapping a frequent observation on expiratory CT images of patients with sarcoid?

C A S E 1 3 9

Sarcoidosis

1. Axial (peribronchovascular).

2. Sarcoidosis, lymphangitic carcinomatosis, lymphoma, and Kaposi's sarcoma.

3. Sarcoidosis.

4. Yes.

Reference

Hansell DM, Milne DG, Wilsher ML, Wells AU: Pulmonary sarcoidosis: morphologic associations of airflow obstruction at thin-section CT. *Radiology* 209:697, 1998.

Cross-Reference

Thoracic Radiology: THE REQUISITES, pp 213–216.

Comment

The inspiratory CT image in the first figure and the expiratory CT image in the second figure demonstrate numerous small lung nodules, which are located predominately in an axial distribution, coursing along the bronchovascular bundles. This distribution of lung nodules is associated with a relatively limited differential diagnosis, including sarcoidosis, lymphangitic carcinomatosis, lymphoma, and Kaposi's sarcoma.

Sarcoid nodules, which represent noncaseating granulomas, are typically perilymphatic in distribution. Such nodules are predominately located along the bronchovascular bundles, radiating from the hila in an axial distribution. Less frequently, the nodules are located in the interlobular septa and subpleural lymphatics, both peripherally and along fissures. Note that several of the nodules in this patient are located peripherally and adjacent to fissures.

The expiratory image in the second figure shows several lobular foci of air trapping, best demonstrated in the left lower lobe posteriorly *(arrow)*. A recent study demonstrated that CT images of patients with sarcoid frequently reveal evidence of small airways disease such as a mosaic pattern of lung attenuation and air trapping on expiratory images. It has been postulated that small airways disease in sarcoid may arise from one of two possible mechanisms: intrinsic granulomas within the small airways and extrinsic peribronchiolar fibrosis.

The combination of airways involvement and interstitial involvement in patients with sarcoidosis may result in heterogeneous patterns of functional impairment on pulmonary function tests. Patients with sarcoidosis may demonstrate a variety of pulmonary function test abnormalities, including restrictive, obstructive, and combined restrictive and obstructive patterns. Interestingly, in the CT study referenced earlier, a reticular pattern of interstitial disease was a stronger predictor of airflow obstruction than CT features of small airways disease.

Notes

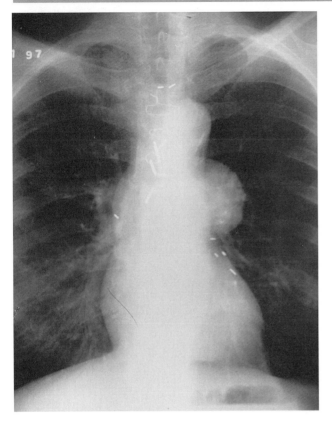

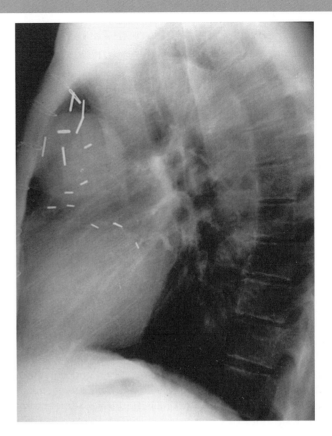

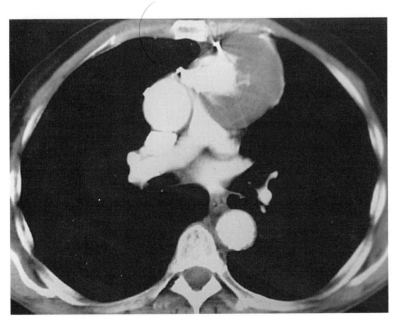

1. This patient's preoperative chest radiograph (not shown) prior to coronary artery bypass graft (CABG) surgery was normal. What is the most likely cause of the anterior mediastinal mass in this case?

2. Is this a common complication?

3. What is the most serious complication of this finding?

4. Is thrombosis a common finding in patients with venous graft aneurysms?

Saphenous Vein Graft Aneurysm Following Coronary Artery Bypass Graft Surgery

1. Aneurysm of a saphenous vein bypass graft.

2. No.

3. Dehiscence of the anastomosis with associated life-threatening hemorrhage.

4. Yes, approximately one half of such aneurysms are partially thrombosed.

Reference

Trop I, Samson L, Cordeau M, Leblanc P, Therasse E: Anterior mediastinal mass in a patient with prior saphenous vein coronary artery bypass grafting. *Chest* 115:572–576, 1999.

Cross-Reference

Thoracic Radiology: THE REQUISITES, pp 431–439.

Comment

The chest radiograph shown in the first and second figures demonstrates a well-circumscribed anterior mediastinal mass located to the left of midline, in close proximity to surgical sutures related to the CABG procedure. The presence of an anterior mediastinal mass in a patient who has undergone CABG should raise the suspicion of an aneurysmal venous graft. The diagnosis can be confirmed with contrast-enhanced CT or MRI. The contrast-enhanced CT image in the third figure confirms the diagnosis of an aneurysm that contains a large amount of peripheral thrombus.

Aneurysms of saphenous vein grafts are a rare but serious complication of CABG. False aneurysms, which are characterized by a disrupted vessel wall, are more common than true aneurysms, which are characterized by an intact vessel wall. False aneurysms are most commonly located at the anastomotic sites. They are typically encountered weeks to months following the procedure. Such aneurysms have been described in association with wound infection, intrinsic weakness of the graft wall, and iatrogenic trauma to the vein during harvesting.

In contrast, true aneurysms are identified most commonly within the body of the graft. Although they may be seen as early as 2 months after surgery, they usually present late in the postoperative period, 5 years or more following surgery. True aneurysms are thought to arise due to progressive atherosclerosis related to exposure of saphenous vein grafts to systemic blood pressure.

Venous graft aneurysms are often asymptomatic and discovered as an incidental finding on routine chest radiographs. When symptomatic, patients generally present with symptoms of myocardial ischemia. Complications of venous graft aneurysms include myocardial infarction, fistula formation to the right atrium or right ventricle, and rupture and secondary hemorrhage. Treatment includes resection of the aneurysm and myocardial revascularization.

Notes

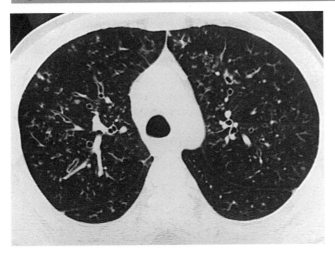 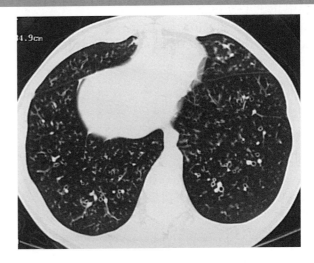

1. In an HIV-positive patient, are these CT findings typical of PCP?

2. What do the centrilobular branching and nodular opacities shown in the figures represent?

3. What two types of infections are most likely?

4. What is the most common type of pulmonary infection to occur in HIV-positive patients—*Pneumocystis*, bacterial, or mycobacterial?

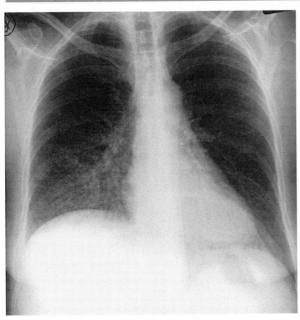

1. This patient underwent renal transplantation 2 months ago and now presents with low-grade fever and nonproductive cough. What is the most common viral pneumonia to occur in solid organ transplant recipients?

2. Is PCP a common opportunistic infection in transplant recipients?

3. What are the characteristic microscopic features of cytomegalovirus (CMV)?

4. With what agents is this infection treated?

Infectious Small Airways Disease in Acquired Immunodeficiency Syndrome

1. No.

2. Impacted bronchioles.

3. Bacterial and mycobacterial.

4. Bacterial.

Reference

McGuinness G: Changing trends in the pulmonary manifestations of AIDS. *Radiol Clin North Am* 35:1029–1082, 1997.

Cross-Reference

Thoracic Radiology: THE REQUISITES, p 398.

Comment

The HRCT images reveal numerous small, branching and nodular centrilobular opacities, consistent with bronchiolitis. There is also mild bronchial dilation and bronchial wall thickening. The findings are consistent with infectious airways disease. In recent years, infectious bronchiolitis and bronchitis have been increasingly recognized in HIV-positive patients. Interestingly, HIV-positive patients also have an increased prevalence of bronchiectasis.

Chest radiograph findings may include bronchial wall thickening and scattered small nodular opacities, the latter representing impacted bronchioles. A symmetric lower lobe predominance is often observed. Isolated small airways disease may be quite difficult to diagnose by conventional radiography because findings are often subtle and may mimic an interstitial pattern. The HRCT features of small airways disease are characteristic and include small (2- to 4-mm) centrilobular branching opacities and nodules, which represent bronchioles impacted with inflammatory secretions. The branching opacities represent bronchioles in profile (oriented in the plane of the transverse CT image), whereas the nodules represent bronchioles in cross section (oriented perpendicular to the image). The term *tree-in-bud* has been used to describe this characteristic appearance. In an HIV-positive patient, this pattern is most closely associated with bacterial and mycobacterial infections. It is only rarely associated with PCP.

Notes

Cytomegalovirus Pneumonia in an Organ Transplant Recipient

1. CMV.

2. No—it is rarely observed due to widespread prophylaxis and occurs primarily in those who are noncompliant with prophylaxis regimens.

3. Cellular enlargement and intranuclear inclusion bodies.

4. Antiviral therapy, foscarnet, or ganciclovir.

References

McGuinness G, Gruden JF: Viral and *Pneumocystis carinii* infections of the lung in the immunocompromised host. *J Thorac Imaging* 14:25–36, 1999.

Conces DJ: Pulmonary infections in immunocompromised patients who do not have acquired immunodeficiency syndrome: a systematic approach. *J Thorac Imaging* 13:234–246, 1999.

Cross-Reference

Thoracic Radiology: THE REQUISITES, pp 140, 141.

Comment

Following renal transplantation, patients are at risk for a variety of infections due to the effects of immunosuppressive therapy. A knowledge of the interval between transplantation and the development of pulmonary infections can help you predict the types of organisms that are likely to cause pulmonary infections.

During the first month following transplantation, the immunosuppressive agents have not yet had a profound effect on the patient's immune system. Opportunistic infections are unusual during this period. Infections are usually caused by organisms that are typically encountered in patients with normal immunity after surgery, particularly gram-negative organisms, and commonly occur due to aspiration or wound catheter-related infections.

Immunosuppression is usually most severe during the second, third, and fourth months following renal transplantation. T-cell mediated immunity is most severely depressed, placing patients at highest risk for viral and fungal infections. CMV is the most common viral agent to affect these patients. Radiographs may show a reticular or nodular pattern and, less commonly, consolidation and discrete lung nodules and masses.

After the fourth month, the immunosuppression regimen is gradually tapered. As the patient's immune system recovers, the organisms that most commonly produce pneumonia in this period are those responsible for most community-acquired pneumonias, such as *Streptococcus pneumoniae*. Because immunosuppressive agents are tapered but not discontinued, patients continue to remain at risk for opportunistic infections, particularly fungal organisms.

Notes

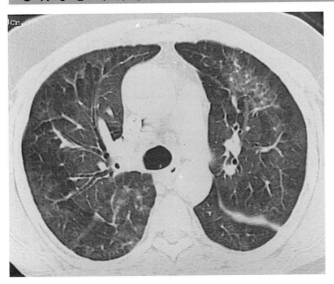 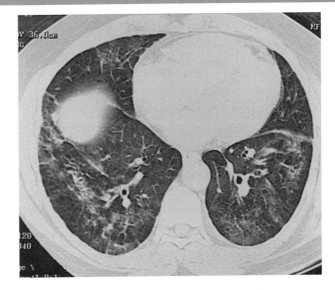

1. This patient has severe pulmonary artery hypertension, pulmonary edema, and a normal pulmonary venous wedge pressure. What is the most likely diagnosis for this triad of findings?

2. Is this disorder associated with a favorable prognosis?

3. In this disorder, which vessels (veins or arteries) are usually enlarged and which are of normal caliber?

4. What is the cause of venous occlusion in this disorder?

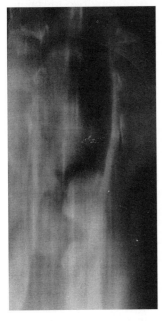 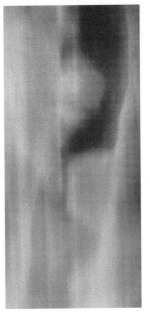

1. What two conditions are most likely to present with multiple tracheal masses?

2. How can MRI help distinguish amyloid from other causes of tracheal masses?

3. This patient also had laryngeal lesions (not shown). Which diagnosis is most likely?

4. What virus is associated with this condition?

C A S E   1 4 3

Pulmonary Venoocclusive Disease

1. Pulmonary venoocclusive disease.

2. No.

3. Enlarged central pulmonary arteries and normal-caliber veins.

4. Intimal fibrosis.

Reference

Swensen SJ, Tashjian JH, Myers JL, et al: Pulmonary venoocclusive disease: CT findings in eight patients. *AJR Am J Roentgenol* 167:937–940, 1996.

Cross-Reference

Thoracic Radiology: THE REQUISITES, p 404.

Comment

Pulmonary venoocclusive disease is a rare disorder that is characterized by obstruction of the pulmonary veins and venules by intimal fibrosis. Increased resistance to pulmonary venous drainage results in pulmonary artery hypertension. The classic triad associated with this condition includes severe pulmonary artery hypertension, radiographic evidence of pulmonary edema, and a normal wedge pressure. Affected patients typically present with symptoms of orthopnea, progressive dyspnea, fatigue, and syncope.

The etiology of this disorder is unknown, but it has been described in association with viral infection, environmental toxins, chemotherapy, radiation injury, contraceptives, and intracardiac shunts. A genetic predisposition has also been reported. There is no effective treatment for venoocclusive disease, and it is usually fatal within a few years of diagnosis. Recently, lung transplantation has been proposed as a potential therapy.

Swensen and associates have reviewed the CT imaging findings in eight patients with this rare disorder. The most commonly observed CT findings were smoothly thickened septal lines, multifocal regions of ground-glass opacity, pleural effusions, enlarged central pulmonary arteries, and pulmonary veins of normal caliber. In the figures, note the presence of numerous thickened septal lines, multiple foci of ground-glass attenuation, slight enlargement of the segmental pulmonary arteries (increased arterial-bronchial ratio), as well as a small left pleural effusion. In the proper clinical setting, these findings are suggestive of pulmonary venoocclusive disease. A definitive diagnosis requires lung biopsy.

Notes

C A S E   1 4 4

Tracheal Papillomatosis

1. Papillomatosis and amyloid.

2. Amyloid demonstrates characteristic low signal intensity on both T1W and T2W sequences.

3. Papillomatosis.

4. Human papillomavirus.

Reference

Gruden JF, Webb WR, Sides DM: Adult-onset disseminated tracheobronchial papillomatosis: CT features. *J Comput Assist Tomogr* 18:640–642, 1994.

Cross-Reference

Thoracic Radiology: THE REQUISITES, pp 358, 362.

Comment

This patient presented with large airway obstruction. Conventional chest radiographs (not shown) revealed multiple tracheal masses. Additional imaging evaluation included conventional tracheal tomograms, shown in the figures. These images reveal the presence of multiple, cauliflower-like masses extending into the tracheal lumen. This patient also underwent laryngoscopy, which revealed several sessile laryngeal lesions. The presence of laryngeal and tracheal lesions is most suggestive of papillomatosis.

Laryngeal papillomatosis is an uncommon condition characterized by the presence of multiple squamous papillomas within the larynx. This disorder is seen primarily in children. Extension of the disease into the trachea and bronchi is referred to as tracheobronchial papillomatosis and occurs in roughly 5% of cases. Isolated tracheobronchial disease is seen more frequently in adults than in children. Rarely, there is dissemination into the lung parenchyma.

The radiologic manifestations of papillomatosis include multiple wart-like and larger cauliflower-like growths projecting into the airway. CT typically shows diffuse nodularity of the airway. Larger lesions, as shown in this case, are less frequently observed. On MRI, the lesions demonstrate intermediate signal intensity, which contrasts with the characteristic low signal intensity associated with amyloidosis. When the lung parenchyma is involved, you may observe centrilobular opacities, nodules, and cavities.

Presenting symptoms depend on the site of involvement. Laryngeal involvement frequently results in hoarseness. Tracheobronchial involvement is associated with symptoms of stridor, wheezing, hemoptysis, and recurrent infections. In children with isolated laryngeal involvement, spontaneous remission is commonly observed. With airway involvement distal to the larynx, however, spontaneous remission is less common.

Notes

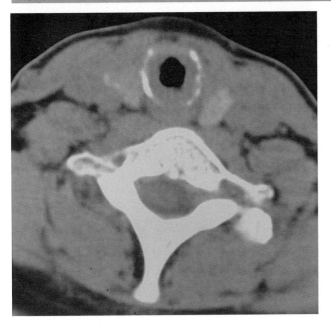
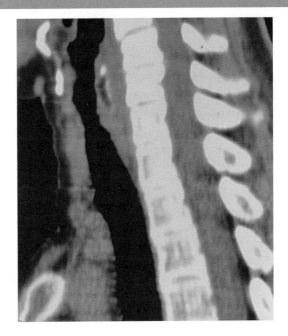

1. List at least five causes of tracheal stenosis.
2. What is the difference between tracheal stenosis and tracheomalacia?
3. Is idiopathic laryngotracheal stenosis more common in men or women?
4. Name at least two nonsurgical treatment options for this condition.

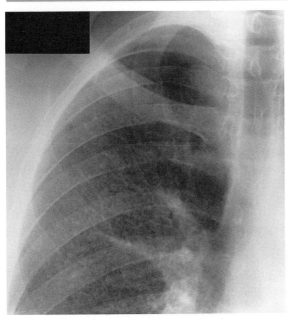
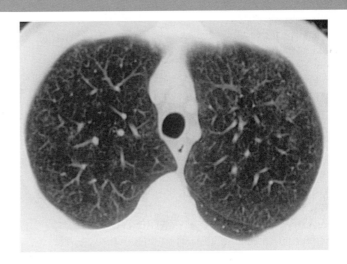

1. Are normal bronchioles usually visible on CT scan images?
2. Name the term that is used to describe nodular and linear branching centrilobular opacities due to small airways disease.
3. Is this pattern pathognomonic for TB?
4. Where in the secondary pulmonary lobule are bronchioles located?

Idiopathic Tracheal Stenosis

1. Trauma, infection, sarcoidosis, Wegener's granulomatosis, relapsing polychondritis, amyloidosis, tracheobronchopathia osteochondroplastica, and chronic obstructive pulmonary disease.

2. Tracheal stenosis refers to a fixed narrowing; in contrast, tracheomalacia refers to excessive collapsibility of the trachea during expiration.

3. Women.

4. Dilation, stenting, steroid injection, cryotherapy, and electrocoagulation.

Reference

Fraser RS, Colman N, Müller NL, Paré PD: Diseases of the airways. In: *Fraser and Paré's, Diagnosis of Diseases of the Chest*, fourth edition. Philadelphia, WB Saunders, 1999, pp 2033–2035.

Cross-Reference

Thoracic Radiology: THE REQUISITES, pp 350–351.

Comment

The axial CT image in the first figure demonstrates luminal narrowing due to circumferential wall thickening of the proximal trachea. The sagittal 2D reformation image in the second figure shows that the stenosis is limited to a small portion of the cervical trachea.

The patient presented in this case has idiopathic tracheal stenosis. Such patients present with narrowing of the subglottic trachea, often accompanied by laryngeal narrowing, with no history of prior intubation, trauma, infection, or systemic illness. When accompanied by laryngeal involvement, this condition is referred to as idiopathic laryngotracheal stenosis.

This disorder typically affects middle-aged women. Affected patients may present clinically with symptoms of shortness of breath, wheezing, stridor, and hoarseness. The diagnosis is often delayed by approximately 2 years before an accurate diagnosis is made.

The radiologic appearance of this condition is variable. The length of the stenosis may range from 2 to 4 cm in craniocaudad dimension. The affected portion of the airway is often severely narrowed to less than 5 mm in diameter. The margins of the stenotic airway may be smooth and tapered (as in this case) or irregular, lobulated, and eccentric. When tracheal stenosis presents with the latter appearance, a primary tracheal neoplasm is an important diagnostic consideration. There are a variety of surgical and nonsurgical treatment options (as detailed in Answer 4).

Notes

Small Airways Disease (Infectious Bronchiolitis)

1. No—normal bronchioles are below the resolution of CT (and HRCT).

2. Tree-in-bud.

3. No.

4. In the center of the secondary pulmonary lobule, adjacent to the pulmonary artery.

Reference

Collins J, Blankenbaker D, Stern EJ: CT patterns of bronchiolar disease: what is "tree-in-bud"? *AJR Am J Roentgenol* 171:365–370, 1998.

Cross-Reference

Thoracic Radiology: THE REQUISITES, pp 396–399.

Comment

The coned-down image of the right upper lobe from a chest radiograph demonstrates a diffuse, fine nodular pattern with some associated small linear opacities. The CT image demonstrates numerous small nodular and branching linear opacities with a centrilobular distribution. The CT appearance is characteristic of a proliferative bronchiolitis, a pattern that is frequently described as "tree-in-bud" because of its resemblance to a tree budding in springtime.

Although the tree-in-bud pattern was originally described in conjunction with TB, it is by no means pathognomonic for this process. Rather, it may be associated with a wide variety of bronchiolar diseases.

An infectious etiology is most common. Acute infectious bronchiolitis is most frequently associated with respiratory synctial virus, adenovirus, and *Mycoplasma* pneumonia. Other important infectious etiologies include mycobacterial and fungal organisms. Chronic diseases of the airways such as asthma, chronic bronchitis, and bronchiectasis are also commonly associated with this pattern. Other causes of proliferative bronchiolitis include aspiration and diffuse panbronchiolitis. The latter is a chronic disease of unknown etiology that occurs almost exclusively in Asians.

Chest radiographs of patients with minimal small airways disease may be normal. In patients with more extensive disease, you may observe a fine nodular pattern, often accompanied by reticular opacities. CT is helpful in differentiating small airways disease from a true miliary pattern. The latter is characterized by a random distribution of small nodules; in contrast, small airways disease is associated with a centrilobular distribution of small nodular and branching opacities.

Notes

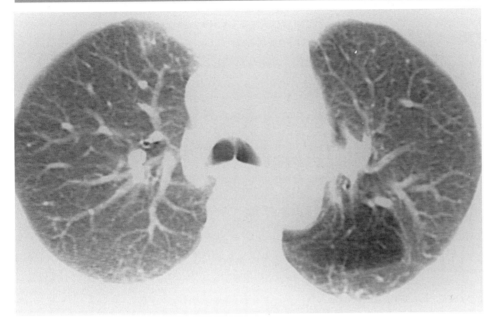

1. Which portion of lung parenchyma is abnormal, the area of increased or decreased lung attenuation?
2. What characteristic allows you to make this distinction?
3. What term is used to describe this pattern of variable lung attenuation?
4. How can you differentiate pulmonary vascular disease from small airways disease as a cause of this pattern?

C A S E   1 4 8

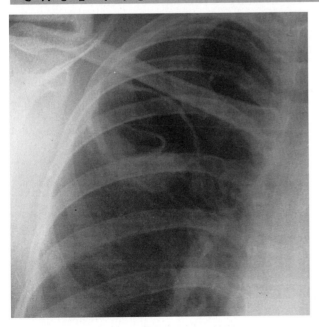

1. What unusual infection is associated with a "cyst within a cyst" as shown in the figure?
2. What term is used to describe the presence of a cyst floating on a fluid level within a larger cyst?
3. Is the lung the most common site of *Echinococcus* cysts?
4. Do these cysts have a predilection for the lower lobes of the lungs?

Mosaic Pattern of Lung Attenuation Secondary to Small Airways Disease

1. Decreased.

2. Fewer and smaller caliber vessels within the low-attenuation area compared with other portions of the lung.

3. Mosaic pattern.

4. Obtain expiratory CT images—only small airways disease demonstrates air trapping.

Reference

Stern EJ, Swensen SJ, Hartman TE, Frank MS: CT mosaic pattern of lung attenuation: distinguishing different causes. *AJR Am J Roentgenol* 165:813-816, 1995.

Cross-Reference

Thoracic Radiology: THE REQUISITES, pp 399-400, 418-419.

Comment

The CT image demonstrates a mosaic pattern of lung attenuation, with a geographically marginated area of low attenuation in the left upper lobe posteriorly. There are several possible causes for a mosaic pattern, including small airways disease, vascular disease, and infiltrative lung disease (producing ground-glass opacification). In the former two entities, the low-attenuation areas are abnormal. In the last entity, the foci of increased attenuation are abnormal.

When you are confronted with a pattern of variable lung attenuation, you should carefully compare the size and number of vessels between the areas of relative low and high attenuation. When the caliber and number of vessels are similar, the areas of relative increased attenuation are abnormal. This appearance is seen in a variety of entities that are characterized by the presence of ground-glass opacities, including acute interstitial infections such as PCP and chronic infiltrative lung diseases. In contrast, a reduction in size and number of vessels within the low attenuation area implies that the low-attenuation foci are abnormal. Such an appearance can be seen in pulmonary vascular disorders, such as chronic pulmonary embolic disease, and small airways disease, such as obliterative bronchiolitis. In cases of small airways disease, the diminished vasculature occurs secondary to reflex vasoconstriction. You can distinguish vascular and small airways etiologies by performing additional expiratory CT scans. Only small airways disease is associated with air trapping on expiratory scans.

Notes

Echinococcus Cysts

1. *Echinococcus*.

2. The water lily sign (also called *sign of the camalote*).

3. No—the liver is most common.

4. Yes.

Reference

Fraser RS, Colman N, Müller NL, Paré PD: Pulmonary infections. In: *Fraser and Paré's Diagnosis of Diseases of the Chest*, fourth edition. Philadelphia, WB Saunders, 1999, pp 1053-1059.

Cross-Reference

Thoracic Radiology: THE REQUISITES, pp 130-131.

Comment

Echinococcus granulosus is the cause of most human forms of hydatid disease. It occurs in two forms: pastoral and sylvatic. The pastoral form is more common. In this form, sheeps, cows, or pigs are the intermediate hosts and dogs are the definitive host. This form of infection is particularly common in the sheep-raising regions of southeastern Europe, the Middle East, Northern Africa, South America, and Australia and New Zealand.

The hydatid cyst contains two layers: an exocyst and an endocyst. Daughter cysts may be formed within the endocyst. The liver is the most common site for echinococcal cysts, accounting for roughly 70% of cysts.

On chest radiographs of patients with *Echinococcus* cysts, you may observe single or multiple well-circumscribed spherical or oval masses. If a cyst communicates with the bronchial tree, air may enter the space between the endocyst and the exocyst, producing a thin crescent of air around the periphery of the cyst. This appearance has been described as the meniscus or crescent sign. When bronchial communication occurs directly into the endocyst, expulsion of the cyst contents may produce an air-fluid level. Once the cyst has ruptured, its membrane may float on the fluid. The term *water lily sign* has been used to describe this characteristic appearance. It is important to know that these characteristic radiographic signs are rarely observed in association with this entity.

When intact, most hydatid cysts are asymptomatic. On cyst rupture there is usually an abrupt onset of cough, expectoration, and fever. Patients may also experience an acute hypersensitivity reaction. Percutaneous aspiration of such cysts has generally not been considered safe owing to the possibility of inciting an allergic reaction or spreading the infection.

Notes

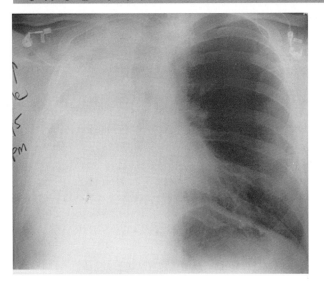
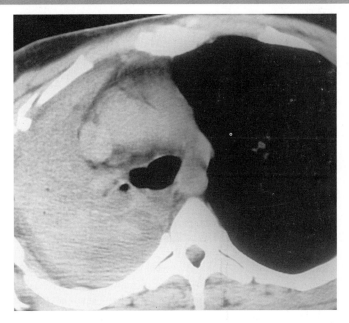

1. Which bronchus is more frequently ruptured, the left or the right?

2. What percentage of cases of acute tracheobronchial injury are associated with a pneumothorax?

3. Rupture of which mainstem bronchus is more commonly associated with pneumomediastinum without pneumothorax?

4. Is bronchial rupture more common than tracheal rupture?

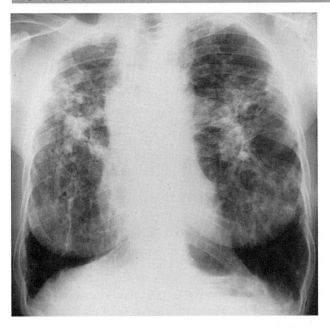

1. Name a sign of upper lobe volume loss present in this case.

2. Name at least two entities that may be associated with conglomerate masses in the upper lung zones.

3. What chronic infiltrative lung disease does chronic berylliosis most closely resemble?

4. Is chronic beryllium disease immunologically mediated?

C A S E 1 4 9

Posttraumatic Bronchial Stricture

1. Right.

2. Approximately 70%.

3. Left mainstem bronchus, because it has a longer mediastinal (extrapleural) course.

4. Yes.

Reference
Stark P: Imaging of tracheobronchial injuries. *J Thorac Imaging* 10:206–219, 1995.

Cross-Reference
Thoracic Radiology: THE REQUISITES, p 179.

Comment
Tracheobronchial injury is an uncommon but serious complication following blunt thoracic trauma. The mainstem bronchi are affected in approximately 80% of cases, followed by the trachea (15%) and distal bronchi (5%). Airway injury is frequently accompanied by upper rib fractures. Note the presence of healing rib fractures in this case, an important diagnostic clue to a traumatic etiology.

Imaging findings can be classified as early and late. Early findings include pneumothorax, pneumomediastinum, and subcutaneous emphysema. Pneumomediastinum without pneumothorax is most common when the mediastinal, extrapleural portion of the airway is ruptured. Pneumothoraces occur in approximately 70% of patients with an airway injury. Such pneumothoraces are typically severe and refractory to chest tube drainage.

In the setting of a complete bronchial rupture, a pneumothorax may be accompanied by the "fallen lung sign." This sign refers to a collapsed lung that sags away from the hilum toward the diaphragm, reflecting its loss of attachment to the hilum.

The diagnosis of tracheobronchial injury is often delayed. Late imaging findings are related to the development of granulation tissue and stricture within the injured bronchus, a process that occurs within 1 to 4 weeks of injury. Late imaging findings include postobstructive atelectasis, pneumonia, abscess, and empyema. The images in this case demonstrate a late presentation of bronchial rupture, manifested by complete collapse of the right lung due to granulation tissue obstructing the injured bronchus.

Notes

C A S E 1 5 0

Chronic Beryllium Disease

1. Cephalad displacement of the pulmonary hila.

2. Silicosis, sarcoidosis, TB, coal worker's pneumoconiosis, and berylliosis.

3. Sarcoidosis.

4. Yes—it represents a cell-mediated hypersensitivity reaction to beryllium bound to tissue proteins.

Reference
Fraser RS, Müller NL, Colman N, Paré PD: Pulmonary diseases caused by inhalation or aspiration of particulates, solids, or liquids. In: *Fraser and Paré's Diagnosis of Diseases of the Chest*, fourth edition. Philadelphia, WB Saunders, 1999, pp 2456–2460.

Cross-Reference
Thoracic Radiology: THE REQUISITES, pp 245–247.

Comment
Chronic beryllium disease (also called *berylliosis*) is a systemic granulomatous disorder caused by exposure to beryllium metal or its salts in the form of dust, fumes, or aerosol. The major sources of occupational exposure include the aerospace and electronics industry, the manufacturing of gyroscopes and nuclear reactors, the processing of ceramics, and the development or handling of beryllium alloys in the manufacturing of airplane landing gear, electronics, and a variety of household appliances. There is typically a delay of 10 to 20 years between exposure and the onset of chronic berylliosis.

Chronic berylliosis is an immunologically mediated disorder that may involve multiple organ systems, including the lungs, lymph nodes, skin, liver, spleen, and bone marrow. The characteristic histologic finding is the epithelioid granuloma, which cannot be distinguished from the noncaseating granuloma of sarcoidosis.

The lungs are the most commonly involved organ system, and exertional dyspnea is a frequent presenting symptom. Radiographic findings in patients with chronic berylliosis are quite similar to those observed in patients with sarcoidosis. Most commonly, you will observe small nodular or reticulonodular opacities, which may involve all three lung zones. Conglomerate masses may also develop. In long-standing disease, you may observe a linear pattern of pulmonary fibrosis that is accompanied by upper lobe volume loss, architectural distortion, and emphysematous bullae. Note these characteristic findings in the figure.

A history of exposure to beryllium can help differentiate this entity from sarcoidosis. Because the imaging and pathologic features are not specific, a diagnosis of chronic berylliosis can be confirmed by a patch test showing hypersensitivity to beryllium. Chronic beryllium disease is treated with steroids. Patients with symptomatic chronic berylliosis have a poor prognosis.

Notes

subpulmonic effusions → elevation of H.D. flattening of HD medially, peaking of H.D. laterally ⇒ get lateral decub.

parapneumonic effusion → effusion 2° bacterial pneumonia (sterile) ⇒ if infected empyema

Loffler's Syndrome → (in DDx peripheral infiltrates.)
(migrating infiltrates. pulmonary infiltrates c̄ eosinophilia)

Castleman's Dz = benign adenopathy

Sympathetic Effusion =

Eosinophillic Granuloma = infiltrative lung dz c̄ cystic pattern

Note: Page numbers in *italics* refer to illustrations.